MIND, BODY, and SOUL
A Guide to Living with Cancer

Nancy Hassett Dahm

MIND, BODY, and SOUL
A Guide to Living with Cancer

By: Nancy Hassett Dahm

Published by:
Taylor Hill Publishing, LTD.
734 Franklin Avenue
PMB 150
Garden City, New York 11530-4525 U.S.A.

Dahm, Nancy Hassett.
   Mind, body, and soul : a guide to living with
cancer / Nancy Hassett Dahm ; editor, Robert F.
Schirmer ; indexer, Frances S. Lennie.-- 1st ed.

   p. cm.
   Includes bibliographical references and index.
   LCCN: 00-134425
   ISBN: 0-9702904-0-3

   1. Cancer--Psychological aspects. 2. Cancer--
Patients--Home care. 3. Cancer--Patients--Pain--
Treatment. 4. Terminal care. 5. Cancer--
Religious aspects. I. Title.

RC263.D34 2000   362.1'96994
                         QBI00-500112

This Book Is Dedicated

To my mother

Letitia Hassett

A mother of pure love, a nurse of perfect compassion, an angel of heaven.

To my husband

Al

This was your vision, my love. This book would not be possible without your wise direction, and constant positive support.

You were my first editor. You never wavered in your mission to help others. You kept me strong and gave me comfort for my soul. This book belongs to you. Be proud my love, you have done a wonderful thing!

Contents

E xperience is the greatest teacher of anything we learn in life, whether it be the experience of a teacher, friend, family member, or one's own life. We are constantly affecting each other by example and by our deeds. We are who we are because of our varied experiences with others. None of us can change or grow without having interactions with others and with our environment. It is appropriate then for me to acknowledge those who contributed to my own experiences, which have allowed me to change and grow as a person and a nurse.

My years at C.W. Post Campus of Long Island University were filled with rich experiences that have directly contributed to the writing of this book. For example, an English assignment — reading Leo Tolstoy's *The Death of Ivan Ilych* — changed forever the way in which I practice nursing. Although written as fiction, Tolstoy's story taught me a truth about the raw anguish and mental suffering that occurs when a person is confronted with serious illness and/or impending death. That simple, seemingly innocuous assignment made me a better nurse.

I credit the entire faculty and staff of my alma mater, Long Island University, with giving me a rich, diversified, and fulfilling education. The years of walking the beautiful grounds helped me heal from the stress of caring for so many people with cancer. The very nature of the campus nurtured my soul. My dedicated professors instilled in me a belief that I could make a difference. My theory on pain management came to me during that time.

Further gratitude is expressed to Dr. David Sprintzen, Professor of Philosophy at C.W. Post Campus of Long Island

University. His brilliance, inspired lectures, and insights have broadened my world and my capability for meaningful thought.

I will always be indebted to George Vossinas, Professor of Anatomy and Physiology at Nassau Community College in New York. His self-discipline, penchant for detail, and relentless commitment to excellence taught me the value of perseverance. His remarkable command of subject matter is attributable to his intellect and to his respect for science, which I have appreciably acquired through his example.

Special appreciation is extended to Maria Machuca, R.N., who first hired me to work in caring for cancer patients. Her constant encouragement and support enabled me to grow professionally and personally. She allowed me to follow my heart.

Thank you, Rabbi Stephen Goodman, for your kind and wise counsel in helping me understand the Jewish perspective of death, dying, and the afterlife. Neither differences in faith or cultural diversity can separate our oneness in humanity. We all seek comfort, reconciliation, and look forward to the world to come.

To Robert Schirmer, my editor, who has been thoughtful, diligent, and exacting in his treatment of this book, I thank you. Your comments and insight were inspirational. You have encouraged my expression to fulfillment.

Teresa Verrastro, my typist, has worked endlessly to help bring this book to fruition. Your labor of love has made me your friend for life.

To my sister, Mary, a fellow nurse, who understands the importance of this work and who has supported me greatly from the beginning, you were my pillar of strength. You have lifted my spirits countless numbers of times. I love you!

Special love and appreciation is felt for my children: Edmar, Tara, Nicholas, and Jeremy. You have allowed me to pursue my studies and career without complaint. In fact, your words of encouragement have given me great confidence. May this book serve as an example for you to see that anything is possible. When you believe in something strongly enough, you must follow your heart.

My deepest respect and gratitude is for my patients, many of whom are in heaven. I was honored and privileged to have been your nurse. Your experiences will profoundly affect me for all the days of my life. You were the greatest teachers of all. You taught me the meaning of life and how precious it is. You taught me about courage and dignity. You showed me what it is to live and die with hope and faith. God bless you all.

The Author is not a doctor. The information contained in this book is for informational/educational purposes only. This information should not be considered to represent the only, or necessarily the best, acceptable or safe method of care or treatment with respect to your own situation or that of your loved one.

Neither this book nor any portion thereof should be considered or construed as medical advice. The book is, rather, a source of information and hope to help you understand and cope with what you are facing, what your doctor is telling you, and most importantly, what options and additional help are available to you. The information contained in this book is general in nature and may not apply in whole or in part to your specific situation.

The drugs/medications and dosages cited are for educational purposes only. Neither the drugs/medications nor the dosages cited may be correct or appropriate in your own situation and could cause serious harm, injury, or death if administered without the advice, consent, and supervision of your physician.

There is no substitute for the advice of your doctor. The author does not recommend any specific drugs/medications, care, or treatment because specific drugs, medications, care, and treatment depend on a variety of factors, such as the patient's age, physical condition, primary and secondary afflictions/diseases, drug interactions and tolerances, etc. A unique and specific course of drugs/medications, care, and treatment must be developed for each individual patient by that patient's physician in conjunction with the patient's medical care team and may be adjusted from time to time by the physician, in accordance with the patient's condition.

The author and publisher make no warranty, guarantee, or other representation, express or implied, as to the validity or sufficiency of any of the information contained in this book. The author and publisher assume no responsibility or liability for any death, injury, and/or damages that may result from the reliance on, use, misuse, misinterpretation, or misapplication of the information contained in this book or in any part or subpart thereof.

Imagine that at a moment, on some day, at no particular time, you or I or someone we love is diagnosed with cancer. This moment changes your or my life forever. Our world is turned upside down as we hurtle through space, disoriented with fear, unable to think clearly. What are we to do first? Who do we turn to? How do we cope?

Imagine now a nurse who has worked with hundreds of people in this situation. A nurse who loves her patients, and has learned from their experiences. A nurse who takes us by the hand and leads us on a journey of discovery, about cancer, what it is, how to live with it, and if necessary, how to die from it. "Mind, Body, and Soul" is such a journey, and Nancy Hassett Dahm is that very nurse. It is a personal journey, informed by her life and her work, enriched by the stories of the people whose lives have touched her. Ultimately it is an inspiring, comforting, and important journey for all of us, no matter who we are or what we do.

For some of us, a cancer diagnosis will mean a series of long and sometimes difficult treatments. It may require having to negotiate systems, and redefining the way that we see ourselves: accepting help from others in ways we never have; being more assertive than we are used to; dealing with changes in our bodies; and coping with feelings of need, embarrassment, and even humiliation.

Some of us will have great success with the treatment, and will continue to live healthy and happy lives for many years to come, while others of us will die. If it becomes clear that we are going to die, how do we do so free of pain, with dignity and love?

As I read this book, I noticed different facets of my identity being called forth. Sometimes I found myself as a doctor, remembering patients I had known in my internship, and wondering whether there was more I could have done for some of them. I remembered the woman who spent several hours describing to me, a 22-year-old medical student, what it was like to be dying. She told me things she had never told anybody, and advised me to enjoy my life, because it passes very quickly. She died that night. At other times I identified as a psychiatrist, reminded of the powerful relationship between our thinking and our bodies. I thought about some of the people who consult me, for example the woman whose mother lives in constant chronic pain from neuropathy. She screams much of the day, which is very stressful for my patient. Until reading this book, I had accepted her doctor's words "there is nothing that can be done for her pain." While reading the first few chapters of the book, I was acutely aware of my role as a concerned and terrified friend. One of my closest friends, Shelley, was writhing in pain on her bed in Southern California, her doctors reluctant to prescribe narcotics. By the time I finished reading the book a couple of weeks later, Shelley had died of disseminated cancer, in an intensive care unit.

Michel Foucault, the French philosopher and historian, said that knowledge and power are inextricable. This inseparability of knowledge and power is most apparent in the health professions where particular expertise rests exclusively in the hands of the professionals. This renders so-called nonexperts disempowered in relation to their own bodies. As Nancy Hassett Dahm tells us, there are doctors who are specifically trained in the art and science of pain management. In the case of my friend Shelley, it was her doctor who ultimately had the knowledge/power to prescribe or not prescribe. He chose not to. I do not know why he left a woman with ovarian cancer suffering throughout Memorial Day weekend. I can only imagine that his choice was guided by what he considered to be in her best interest. I believe this decision was influenced by the powerful discourse in our culture that drugs are addictive and should be avoided if possible. I think as doctors we are afraid of authorities, and do what we can to avoid prescribing strong analgesics. This idea is further strengthened by our cultural narratives about illness, which praise people for having a "high pain threshold," and see them as brave heroes for being stoic and not complaining.

"Mind, Body, and Soul" is an important work. It furnishes us with a vast body of knowledge regarding cancer: living with it, and dying from it. As readers we are empowered to take charge of our own process throughout the course of our illness, or the illness of a loved one. As such, we the "patients" become experts of our own bodies. For doctors this is an important book too. It reminds us to listen to our patients. Nancy Hassett Dahm reminds us that the best way to measure pain is to ask someone whether they have pain, and how severe it is. In the 21st century there is no reason for anyone to suffer in pain, or to die in pain. We have sophisticated technology, pharmaceuticals, and methodologies available to us, to ensure that we can all die with dignity, pain-free, in our homes, should we choose.

I encourage you to read this book with an open mind. While it may be uncomfortable, it is ultimately a book that creates freedom for us; freedom to face our lives and our deaths with information, wisdom, and courage.

Paul Browde, M.D.
Psychiatrist
Faculty, Albert Einstein College of Medicine

Introduction

*I feel I know you very well. You don't know me, but
I have watched you. I have walked your journey
many times before. You don't know me, yet I was
there…Mind, Body, and Soul.*

Nancy Hassett Dahm

I have dealt with the entire spectrum of cancer and its effects on the minds, bodies, and souls of hundreds of cancer patients and their families.

I wrote this book so that you can benefit from the knowledge and experience I have acquired over the years. It contains everything you need to know about living with cancer. It is a guide for everyone: all patients, beginning with the newly diagnosed, and all family members. It is for the cancer patients who will recover and survive and for those who will survive in another way.

For the newly diagnosed cancer patient, I know you have a host of questions you want answered, starting with the most basic: will you get the support you need? Can you trust your doctor to "be there" for you? Will your HMO impose restrictions on your treatment? How will you be able to control your anxiety, stress, and fears? What about pain? Can it be eliminated or controlled? And what about the bigger picture — who are you, deep down? Is there really a soul that is eternal?

Mind, Body, and Soul is an encompassing approach to cancer that will help all of you find the answers to the crucial questions. Just as importantly, it will help you deal with immense difficulties you face. You will learn what can be done to make your lives better. I will answer your questions, discuss choices, and give you the information needed to empower yourself in making decisions that are right for you. I will cover the physical, psychological, and spiritual aspects of cancer and provide solutions that are practical and at times philosophical in nature.

You and your family will journey with me through what lies

ahead. I am going to show you how it is to live with cancer for most people, and how much better it can be for you. Knowledge is strength, after all. I promise I will make you strong.

Our journey begins in the **Valley of the Forgotten** (Chapter 1). It's a place where people encounter terrible indifference. It's a look at how attitudes and behaviors of some physicians, nurses, and family members can affect you. You will read about actual patients I've cared for and how we resolved the problems we encountered. I will always give suggestions in case you find yourself in a similar situation. My goal is to help you recognize that certain attitudes and behaviors are just not acceptable. I don't accept them as a nurse and you shouldn't accept them as a patient. I am preparing you for what you might experience.

A Storm Is Brewing (Chapter 2) is a storm indeed. We journey through the brambles of managed care and what it means to you as a person in need of service. I discuss HMOs, cost of enrollment, criteria for disenrollment, and problems and solutions. Your ability to access care is directly related to the type of insurance you have. This information is highly important to you and your course of treatment.

Through the Forest of Fear (Chapter 3) explains the fears you are likely to have. I give you explanations of what they are. Most often, we fear what we don't know. Once you have the information you need, you are less likely to be fearful. That is why I deal with this subject early in this book. I explain procedures and side effects of some treatments. I discuss the usual nondrug and drug interventions so that you can be knowledgeable and question your physician if a certain treatment for a side effect is appropriate for you.

Overcoming Stress (Chapter 4) is all about how to help yourself calm down. All kinds of practical advice is included here for you to refer to. You can use one or several measures. I talk about deep breathing, massage, mental imagery, humor — they all work very well in keeping you focused on everyday life so you can enjoy the people around you. Overcoming stress is important for you because you face enormous stresses in coping with cancer. The turmoil and treatments of cancer compromise your immune system. It is very important that you get enough rest, sleep, nutrition, and mental peace. You need a strong mind/body/soul connection to keep as strong and healthy as possible. Overcoming stress will help you get in touch with your inner self.

Home Is Where the Heart Is (Chapter 5) explains that, in truth, there is no place like home. It is a refuge and place where you are protected and loved. I explain why people with cancer need to be in their own homes. You and your family will learn about homecare. You'll learn what services can be provided in the home and for how long. I explain medical coverage and cost, as well as the HMO's role and what *not* to expect. As a cancer patient, you could receive homecare (for short duration or longer) depending on the need for professional intervention. You will also learn if you qualify for free hospitalization and/or free medications. You have to plan your care and this chapter will be invaluable in helping you to do that.

A Path Away from Pain (Chapter 6) brings us to one of the book's most important subjects. Seventy-five percent of cancer patients experience pain during the course of illness. You need to know not only why you are having pain, but what you can do about it. Most pain is under-treated because of lack of knowledge and understanding of doctors, nurses, and patients. You will learn how to assess your pain and be your own advocate for pain management. You will have a full understanding of how to keep yourself pain-free.

A Path Away from Pain – the Medications. (Chapter 7) discusses the second half of this subject — pain medications. You will learn what is usually prescribed according to the medical protocols established by experts in pain management. You need to know the different medications and how they are used. The purpose of this chapter is to provide you with enough knowledge so you can speak to your physician when he or she is not helping you manage your pain effectively. This knowledge will actually help your physician prescribe what is best for you. This chapter will also dispel the inbred myths and fallacies associated with taking pain medications for cancer pain.

By now, we will have accomplished a great deal. You will feel stronger and more sure of how to handle your affairs. You will know your rights and possibilities. You will not be a passive recipient of either illness or treatment. You will realize just how much courage you have and what choices are available to you.

A Rest in the Field of the Philosophs (Chapter 8) is the perfect time and place to take a journey through mental imagery. We are now transported back through the centuries to hear the words of Socrates, Plato, and Marcus Aurelius. It is here where you may find the meaning of life, self, and the soul. It is here where you can rest and realize that your questions were also the questions of the great thinkers of the past. Now their questions become your answers. You'll see how we all question our mortality. The field is a place to meditate on the broader possibilities of mind, body, and soul. After a long deserved rest, you will be ready for some good news.

In **Now Climb the Hills of Hope** (Chapter 9), you will see all the hopeful things that are happening to improve the quality of your care and life. You will learn about some of the most advanced research and diagnostic methods for detecting and treating cancer. You will learn about clinical trials, new drugs, and technological advances.

To the Mountain of Visions (Chapter 10) brings you to the edge of the unexplained. Miracles and things divine do happen and you will be comforted by accounts of patients, families, and my own personal experiences. There is a bridge between the seen and the unseen world. It's all about possibilities. Miracles happen. The unexplained happens. When you keep hope alive, anything can happen.

Heaven Is Waiting (Chapter 11). This special last chapter is for families who need help and instructions on what to do when a loved one is dying. We will work together to bring the most care and comfort we can give. This is the most sacred time in a person's life and this time should hold a special meaning for all of us. Care is your greatest and final gift to your loved one. Be confident that you'll do fine. We all must die. It may be later rather than sooner for most, but know this: death deserves as much respect as life. And what we fear most just might be what we should fear least. This is where the hope of mankind continues into the realm of possibilities.

Now you see where we are going. Do not take this journey alone. You need to be with someone who has experience in the matters that concern you: there is too much to hope for and too much of life left for all of you to enjoy. I want you to live your life with meaning and look at everything as if you were seeing it for the first time. We have a lot to do, and you will be made stronger for having walked this way with me.

Chapter One
Valley of the Forgotten

Be not ashamed to be helped; for it is thy business to do thy duty like a soldier in the assault on a town. How then, if being lame thou canst not mount upon the battlements alone, but with the help of another it is possible?

Marcus Aurelius Antoninus

There is a purpose to everything in life. I believe that now. I thought I became a nurse to make a living. It became much more than that. Looking back, I realize it was no accident that I was hired for a hospice team. While I had no prior experience with caring for cancer patients, the idea was comfortable to me. I thought I could just blend in and help out. That was not the case. My first year in hospice was the most difficult year of my life. It tore at the very core of who I was as a person and a nurse. A whirlwind of grief surrounded me. I cried for six months. I went to many wakes with a feeling of failure and helplessness, sitting in the back, viewing my patient from a distance. I wondered what could have been done to make it easier for him or her. The lessons I learned would benefit my next patient. That was my promise.

There were many promises that year. I could have walked away and gone on to other areas where nurses managed fractured hips, congestive heart failures, and so on, where almost everyone survives. I didn't. My caseload of 35 to 50 patients primarily had a prognosis of less than six months to live; and the average survival time was two months by the time I received them. That "fight or flight" feeling of anxiety was constantly with me. Courage came to me when there were good outcomes. A good outcome was when a patient died pain-free and surrounded by a caring family. It was hard work to achieve that kind of an outcome. It took everything I had and everything the patient had. And the more I learned, the stronger I became. It was the year of my metamorphosis.

Then things really began to change. There were more and more people who were having good outcomes. Ninety percent of my patients died pain-free. There are some health care professionals who feel that dying with dignity is an illusion or myth. I am here to tell you that is not so. I have had over 400 patients and most of them found themselves, came to terms with their mortality, had quality of life, enjoyed freedom from pain, and died with dignity. These are the people I pulled out of the "Valley of the Forgotten."

Let me describe this valley and then guide you away from it so you can take control and find the path toward emotional and physical peace.

The Valley of the Forgotten is a place of indifference, pain, grief, and abandonment. Because of our society's desensitization to death and dying, and even illness, indifference has become a commonplace attitude among health care professionals and society at large. We see this in our everyday contact with people.

I believe there are common behaviors and attitudes facing all cancer patients, from the moment of diagnosis, through the course of treatment, and during the convalescent period. There will be encounters with people who are insensitive. This will be more evident and irritating to you now because you will be dependent on many people for your care. It comes with the territory of being sick and needing the help of everyone from secretarial staff to nurses, physicians, technicians, and others. Simply put, not everyone will be kind, understanding, or even courteous. Given all of the above, it is not surprising that pain is still very much a part of being ill in this country. Only lately have there been unified, organized efforts to eradicate it as a necessary by-product of surgery or disease.

Grief comes not only with having been given a diagnosis of cancer, but also in the possible loss of all that you have treasured in this world. This includes the loss of self-respect you feel because of the indifference and insensitivity of others towards you. Thus, you have feelings of being abandoned at the very time you need people most. For many people, this is the worst part of being ill.

I will now give you a view of why the attitudes I have described exist. Keep in mind that not all physicians, nurses, or families are like this. For our purposes here, it is important to show you attitudes and behaviors that are not in anyone's best interest.

Physicians and the Cancer Patient

The physician in our society is trained in objective science. His or her goal is to cure an illness or disease. Developing an emotional attachment to a patient is not taught or encouraged in medical schools. In addition, the physician has his or her own belief system and culture that may influence how he or she cares for you, the patient. The physician's personal feelings about death, for instance, may prevent him or her from being able to discuss it with you. And there is often a sense of failure in admitting there is nothing more that can be done. The resulting behavior can be avoidance of the patient. Studies have shown, for example, that most physicians choose not to tell the patient when he or she has a terminal illness. And most do not discuss the prognosis, even when directly asked, because they fear the patient's response. But in studies done over the years, most patients have said that they would prefer to be told the truth about their diagnosis.

Medical schools are now trying to provide students with a multicultural approach to medicine and are incorporating sensitivity training, but unfortunately the students aren't really interested. They are not taking these elective courses because they take valuable time away from mainstream medical studies. Doctors who place academics above compassionate, sensitive care miss the point because care given without compassion is not care at all. It's just academics with indifference.

I have observed that physicians are very good at handling emergencies and trauma because they're involved in short-term action and they are in control. I believe they are not good at the long-term process of managing a patient who has a potentially terminal illness because, in addition to the factors discussed above, it basically involves their losing control, and because they are confronted with emotions they don't know how to deal with.

A case in point: I had a patient with recurrent lung cancer that had metastasized. I'll call her Ruth. She was very thin. She experienced nausea and pain, and complained of being very cold all the time. I could also see that her anxiety level was "through the roof." Ruth and her husband were outraged. She had seen her oncologist, whose only comment was, "we can't have you in a fur-lined bikini this summer, you have to eat more." No medications or other suggestions were given. When I called the oncologist for anti-anxiety medication, she told me, "that's not my field." When I called her cardiologist, he said "that's not my field, I only take care of the heart."

I explained to the patient and her husband that she needed a doctor who would take responsibility for her needs. They agreed. I called another physician, gave a case history, and Ruth had the medication she needed that night. She then went to see her new physician the next day. Of course, I spent a lot of time teaching her how to take control of her care, what to eat, how to manage pain, and how to relax. We also worked on trust issues. She improved considerably. One reason for her improvement was that she no longer felt abandoned. She had a whole new team of doctors who were responsive to her needs. The other reason for improvement was that her hope was renewed. When there is renewed hope, there is a change in how you live each day.

In Ruth's case, there was such a radical change that she was discharged from my services shortly thereafter. Recently, I was sitting with my husband in a local restaurant when I noticed a woman waiting for a table. It was Ruth. I sat with her and her husband as they waited for their meal. She was cheerful and had a wry sense of humor. We laughed and held hands. It was great to see her enjoy life. What made this so special was that she had been given a two-month prognosis five months earlier. Three months past her "due time," she was eating steak and driving a car.

Generally speaking, physicians are not well trained in

managing pain. Their general belief is that pain is normal. As a result, they do not prescribe pain medications that the patient needs because they don't know what medications are available or in what dosages to prescribe them. For these reasons, the American Pain Society and the World Health Organization have established guidelines and protocols on how to prescribe pain medication and how much to give. The problem is that most physicians don't know these protocols exist. Eight out of ten of my 400 patients did not have the proper symptom control when they first came into hospice care. I had to fight for every change in pain medication. Suddenly, I'd be on my feet in an attempt to make a point to a physician (a point he or she couldn't see, nor did they care to). Most times, the doctor would concede. If a physician refused, I'd suggest that the family find another who would be more receptive and responsible. Fortunately, there are many physicians who <u>do</u> care and are knowledgeable about pain medication. Some are internists and some are oncologists. Chances are, someone you know may know one.

A case in point: I had a patient whom I will call Louis. He was in a lot of pain. Louis had pain levels of 8 to 10 on the 0-10 scale (this will be covered in a later chapter). His pain was causing depression, lack of sleep, agitation, inability to eat properly, and a general feeling of hopelessness. Every time he went to the clinic, he saw a different doctor. His pain medication was changed often, with a morphine drug being replaced with a non-morphine drug. I went to the clinic and asked one of the physicians if he would take primary responsibility for handling Louis's pain management. He said he would. A note was placed on his chart that only Dr. Smith was to order pain medications for Louis. We put a pain scale flow sheet in the house and Dr. Smith managed his pain according to the pain scale ratings. Everyone in the household, including the home health care aide, was instructed on how to use it.(You will also be trained in the use of a pain scale flow sheet in Chapter 6.) Louis remained practically pain-free for the remainder of his time.

You have rights as a human being and as a patient. You

have the right to be respected. You shouldn't have to ask for that. You have the right to be told the truth, if you want it, because in truth there is potential for healing. You have the right to compassionate care, because in love all things are possible. And you have the right to be pain-free, because it is possible and it is our obligation as health professionals to make you as comfortable as possible.

Here are some suggestions for dealing with physicians:

- You need to sit down with the physician and explain to him or her that you want to be told the truth, if this is how you feel. A conspiracy of silence is far more threatening to your well-being.

- Discuss options with the doctor with regard to chemotherapy, radiation, and/or other treatments.

- Ask to be referred to a pain specialist if you are having pain that your doctor cannot manage effectively. (Pain management will be discussed in Chapters 6 and 7.)

- If you are not currently under the care of an oncologist, you should be. If you find that he or she is not right for you, find another.

- You should always get a second opinion.

- Seek treatment in a hospital that specializes in cancer treatment.

Nurses and the Cancer Patient

The professional nurse has a responsibility to protect the patient from harm. The nurse's duty is to evaluate the patient's physical condition and assess any environmental factors that may impact negatively on the patient. This includes living conditions, family dynamics and relationships, and psychological and physical adaptations. Most nurses practice in their area of interest. That is to say that nurses who take care of the general adult population are not especially equipped to care for cancer patients. This is a special field with its own standards of focus. While the general practice nurse will tend to focus on the patient's physical condition, the oncology nurse will assess the patient's physical, psychological, and spiritual needs in depth. The oncology nurse is well-educated in the many issues, studies, and protocols in caring for the cancer patient.

That said, the nurse may be having her or his own difficulties in dealing with a cancer patient. Like physicians, nurses also bring their belief systems and culture to their practice. While we are trained to focus on the patient's background and beliefs, we unfortunately can let our own values dictate how we respond.

A case in point: I had a patient whom I will call Frank. It was established from the beginning that Frank wanted to die at home. He had lung cancer and had been in hospice care for about a year. His condition was deteriorating. He had an ulcer that required the nurse to see him on a daily basis for wound care. He also needed oxygen. The nurse was a general practice nurse who took good care of him. We all supported Frank and his wife, who had been getting regular visits from the social worker for coping skills and relaxation techniques. Everything was going well until there was an abrupt change in Frank's condition, which should have been expected given the progression of the disease. It wasn't anything that couldn't have been handled in the home. The nurse panicked, which led the wife and patient to panic, and they were all arguing over whether to call 911. My attempts to calm the nurse and the family failed. The ambulance was called and the patient was taken to the hospital, where he died a few days later. That's just what the patient and his wife didn't want.

As professionals, we have to respect what the patient wants, not what we want. The consequence of the above story is that Frank's wife will remember the turmoil of that day more than she will remember the relative peace they had all year, and she will always regret that she wasn't there when he died. If Frank had had an oncology nurse instead of a general practice nurse, there would have been no panic and Frank would have died at home.

When I train nurses on caring for patients like Frank and Louis, I always say, "the decisions we make today not only affect today, but can reach thirty or more years into the future, because families will always remember how their loved one died."

Putting the issue of specialization aside for a moment, I believe most nurses love their patients. They are experts in the art of caring. Unfortunately, due to constraints in insurance and cost- effective measures by many home care agencies, nurses have little time to spend with patients. Because of insurance, home visits have been cut to an absolute minimum, and because of cost reduction needs, nurses have to see many patients in a day. This leaves you with a nursing visit that is "short, sweet and to the point." Quality of care suffers and so do you.

Here are some suggestions for obtaining the best nursing care in the home care situation:

- Write any questions down that you may want to ask.

- The nurse should write the answers down for you. Ask her or him to do that.

- Report problems with pain, nausea, vomiting, loss of appetite, anxiety, sleep disturbances, dizziness, shortness of breath, difficulty urinating or moving bowels.

- In the case of terminal illness, tell the nurse what you want: Do you want to stay at home? Do you want to be referred to hospice care? (Hospices are designed to give you full medical team care in your home.)

- Ask the nurse if you can have a social worker. They are specialists in helping you cope with your disease, and can help with on financial entitlements, and community services.

- If you still have pain and the doctor hasn't changed the frequency of the medication or the medication itself, ask to speak with the nursing supervisor of the home care agency. She should call your doctor and advocate on your behalf. (I will show you in Chapter 6 how you can be your own advocate.)

- Discuss with your nurse your wishes for a health care proxy and advance directives. (These will be explained fully in chapter 5.) This is to ensure that your decisions regarding what medical procedures you want done (and those you want withheld) will be followed.

The Family

When the crisis of a deteriorating condition occurs, family dynamics can become complex. Each member of a family may react in a different manner, or they may react the same. Each behavior manifested by the patient can have a different effect on each member of the family. Actually, every stage the patient goes through, the family usually goes through also. But the stages may occur at different times!

Families seek equilibrium. If equilibrium is threatened by a life-threatening illness of a member, then there is crisis and stress. For our purposes here, I will talk about responses that threaten the family's unity and affect the outcome of care in the home.

In 1969, Dr. Elizabeth Kubler-Ross presented a framework for the stages of death: denial, anger, bargaining, depression, and acceptance. These are normal adaptation responses by the patient and the family. They are also the stages that patients and families go through when there is a diagnosis of cancer. They do not necessarily occur in that order, and some family members may exhibit depression while another has anger, and still another may be in denial, and so on. These adaptive responses, while normal, have an effect on how the family and patient progress towards resolution. The problem is that resolution may not happen unless the patient and family openly communicate with each other.

What is feared most by the cancer patient is the fear of being abandoned. An example of a maladaptive response is avoidance behavior, where the family isolates the sick or dying person in a room that is dark, rarely visits him or her, and rarely communicates except when bringing food or medication, etc. Avoidance behaviors are used as defense mechanisms. The person who is ill may have anger and hostility toward the family members, which fosters continued avoidance on their part. The anger could come from loss of control, loss of her or his family role, and anger with impending death. What invariably happens with a family that uses avoidance is that shared grief, reconciliation, and shared love does not occur. The patient dies alone and the family is left with unresolved grief and guilt.

The family is the patient's last line of defense and protection. Families are generally distrustful of anyone coming from the outside and entering their home. Think about it. You're uncomfortable when a repairman comes. You become tense. "Just fix the problem and leave" is what you're thinking. When he does leave, it's a relief. This is because your home is the boundary line that separates you from the rest of society and people need permission to invade your space.

In the context of a serious illness, this presents a unique problem because caregivers need time to do their work effectively. That means you and your family will need to overcome the tension and stress of having strangers in your home. During your illness there may be a need for a nurse, aide, social worker, and physical therapist to be in your home several times a week. Your schedule is disrupted; people may not arrive on time, or may not show up. This leads to anger, distrust, anxiety, and other negative feelings.

As caregivers, our only access to the patient is through the family. If we don't have the family's permission to work with everyone, then communication breaks down and we can't provide total care — of the patient and the family. Total care involves counseling for the patient and family in coping skills, discussing fears, and giving guidance in how to express that which is most uncomfortable. It involves the physical care of the patient and maintaining the highest level of comfort and happiness they can achieve.

The one major difficulty experienced by the patient and family is coping with the stress. The stress factor separates people and causes them to fraction off emotionally in different directions. Stress blocks communication and comprehension. Stress among family members creates anxiety, depression, fear, sleeplessness, inability to eat, weight loss, and disruptive behavior like anger, hostility, and avoidance. It is only when the stress is relieved that we can all carry out our roles and serve a mutual purpose in giving what your loved one and our patient needs most...a calm, quiet, comfortable place in which to be cared for.

Suggestions for relieving stress:

- Recognize that feelings of anger, despair, and confusion are normal reactions to a diagnosis of cancer.

- Take one day at a time. Don't try to look too far into the future.

- Sit down as a family and openly discuss your feelings. Keep no secrets from each other. Time is too precious.

- Make a plan: As a family, discuss treatment options with the physician. Your plan should involve the loved one's greatest needs. Assess your financial reserves. Work out travel arrangements for medical appointments.

- Learn all you can about the type of cancer involved. The more you know, the better equipped you'll be to ask questions and make decisions.

- Use all the resources available to you. (Resources are listed in the Appendix section of this book.)

- Use your community for supportive services, including your place of worship and your local hospitals, which can put you in touch with specialists, nutritionists, home care agencies, hospice care, and transportation services from the community.

- Try to enjoy your life with the things you like most; music, reading, walking, gardening, being with animals, relatives, and friends.

- Talk of love, think of happiness, and use humor. Humor is very good medicine. Humor increases your immune response, helps alleviate stress, and serves to improve your overall well-being.

- Start now to make your own decisions. There is power in self direction. You will feel more "in control" of your life.

To summarize, we've learned that attitudes and behaviors of physicians, nurses, and families have an effect on the quality of care delivered and can have a significant emotional impact on the patient. You want to avoid any breakdown in communication resulting from people acting independently of each other rather than in an interdependent relationship. Poor outcomes in home care are a result of poor communication: The patient in pain doesn't insist on pain management because he doesn't communicate that to the doctor. Why? Because he doesn't know it is possible, and because he doesn't know how to ask for it. You will learn how to communicate that need to your doctor.

The nurse who panicked by calling 911 was not communicating with her patient as to his wish that he remain at home. It could have been a peaceful passing. We constantly have to remind ourselves of what the patient wants. It is our duty to respect those wishes. Would it be what we would want for ourselves when our own time comes? We may not know that until we are faced with it. But in caring for a patient or a loved one, what he or she wants is what counts.

All of us, the doctors, nurses, families, and friends have to be very mindful of the fact that we are caring for a person who has lived a life of value. We cannot be desensitized to a person's feelings, because if we are, we put the person into the Valley of the Forgotten. And after all, we are talking about your spouse, mother, father, sister, brother or dear friend.

We have much farther to travel, so we best be leaving this place. Although we are traveling the rough roads in the beginning, it will get easier to bear. Be confident that we will overcome these problems as we continue.

Chapter Two
A Storm Is Brewing

The Art of Life is more like the wrestler's art than the dancer's, in respect of this, that it should stand ready and firm to meet onsets which are sudden and unexpected.

Marcus Aurelius Antoninus

My first storm occurred when I was five years old. To this day I still recall it whenever the skies turn dark and forbidding. My sister had taken me on a long walk. The weather was nice and I had no worries as she held my hand. Then, letting go of my hand, she assured me she'd be right back. There I was, a little child protected one moment and lost the next. As my eyes searched for her in panic, I heard a rumbling in the sky; darkness covered the day. I was terror-stricken standing alone as the thunder grew more angry. A hard rain began to fall. Lightning was heading my way and I couldn't move. I was powerless. She eventually returned and laughed saying, "God is just moving furniture in heaven." To this day, when I hear rumblings, I tense with expectation and I'm still afraid.

There are many kinds of storms we have to weather in life. It doesn't get any easier as we age. We are still frightened of being powerless and not knowing where to turn for help.

Our way of life has changed greatly over the past forty years. Our parents never worried about medical bills, and most families were able to get by. The need for a second mortgage to pay medical expenses was unheard of. It's different today. People do worry about bills and yes, people are getting second mortgages to pay for experimental treatments, transplants, and the like.

The Storm that Is Brewing Is Managed Care

Managed care is in every doctor's office, every hospital, and almost every home in America. It touches our lives in a most personal way as we react to the inequitable manner in which most managed care HMOs operate. What do I mean by inequitable? Well, there are denials of referrals to specialists, lifetime caps on benefits, incentives for doctors to provide less care to maximize profits, and "gag clauses" that prohibit doctors from discussing their opinions of the managed care organization they are under contract to serve. There is extreme difficulty in filing a malpractice suit when an HMO's decision has caused injury or death. This goes back to a law established in 1974 which prohibits such a suit. Federal judges are interpreting the law in favor of managed care organizations and cases are being thrown out of court. (This is soon to change.)

It is not without prejudice that I speak of the inequities of such a system. Too often it is poor and middle-class citizens who are lost in a forest of bureaucratic bramble that leaves them without any power or freedom. We have worked by the sweat of our brows to provide for our families. Then, one day, out of nowhere, sickness strikes. Our dream of longevity with our loved ones seems gray. The shock of a life-threatening illness supercedes our ability to think of what to do. Then comes the fear of not being able to pay your way back into life and the fear that your managed care provider will cause your premature death in the interests of cost efficiency.

Take, for example, the case of a 52-year-old man who says his HMO misdiagnosed a brain tumor for two years, then later told him his tumor was inoperable. They refused to pay for treatment. He had to drain his retirement savings to pay all costs of radiation treatments.

Mental Anguish Can Be Greater than Physical Pain

American families are already stretched to their financial limits with both parents working. A storm is brewing and before, or even if, it blows over, it will be far worse than hearing "God move furniture up in heaven." This storm of controversy involving managed care directly affects you and your access to health care. The controversy lies within the dichotomies of principles and ethics surrounding the managed care system. For example: cost versus quality, control versus freedom of choice, financial incentives to the doctors for non-referrals versus welfare of the patient, and denial of care versus right to appeal to an unbiased third party are all major issues of controversy.

Many years of abuse and fraud have cost the Federal Government billions of dollars and has depleted the Medicare Trust Fund to the verge of bankruptcy. The practice of double billing, overcharging, phantom billings, unnecessary and/or lengthy hospitalizations and tests, etc. have all led us into the age of managed care.

To illustrate the problem, let's look at the case of one of my cancer patients, who had a prognosis of two weeks to live. Her insurance was Medicare. She was being well cared for by her husband, who took great pains in ensuring her comfort. Pain was not an issue until one night she developed severe pain. She was taken to the hospital solely for pain management, but they proceeded with surgery on a non-cancerous organ, performed a cardiac catheterization, did CT and MRI Scans, a blood transfusion, intubation, and finally put her on a respirator when she developed breathing difficulty. These actions were totally unnecessary procedures for a person with two weeks to live. Her last week of life was spent with her hands tied down to the bed and she was kept sedated so as to prevent her from fighting the intubation tube. The pain and trauma she endured was hardly justified. She was sent from this world with the most blatant disregard. Whose interest did it serve? We know it wasn't hers.

But now the pendulum has swung to the opposite extreme and it will take many sacrificial lambs of misfortune to create a better balance in health care that is both cost effective and just.

Years ago, most Americans were in a "fee for service" type of insurance in which 80 percent of doctors' and hospital bills were paid by the insurance company. The remaining 20 percent was paid by the insured in out-of-pocket costs. The patient had freedom of choice of doctors and hospitals and could obtain a second opinion if not satisfied with the first.

This all changed because of rising health care costs. Medicare and Medicaid had been like a green light in heavy traffic. Everyone was speeding ahead to get the most out of their mileage. The cost of national health expenditures in 1990 was $675 billion. Managed care is the red light of regulation with limits on access to care, specialists, and services.

Many of us, including myself, find the complexities of managed care...well, complex. It is here to stay and we had best try to understand it if we are to be our own health care advocates. I'll give you a briefing on what it's all about.

What Is an HMO?

HMO is an acronym meaning health maintenance organization. An HMO functions as both a health insurance company and the provider of care. HMOs have been in operation since 1933, beginning with the Kaiser Plan and the Health Insurance Plan of Greater New York City. Today, managed care and HMOs provide coverage for 85 percent of employed workers in the United States. Managed care is a system that provides and manages health care by regulating the members' use of its services. The health care is delivered by a specific network of doctors and hospitals. The monthly premium is paid by the member or by the employer to the HMO or managed care insurance company. A wide range of services are usually provided with no other out-of-pocket expenses, except for a small co-payment for office visits and medications. Some HMOs use the traditional model, utilizing their own freestanding clinics and hospitals and employing their own staff. Other types of HMOs contract with providers to deliver the service. There are also variations in the HMO model:

Preferred Provider Organizations (PPOs)

This is a network of providers, i.e. physicians, hospitals, and other health care services that contract with a third-party payer (the PPO) on a fixed payment basis. These providers do not necessarily operate out of just one facility. The PPO enrollee receives a list of providers who are in and around their community. A small co-payment for office visits and medication is usually charged.

Point of Service Plan (POS)

The Point of Service Plan offers the insured a choice of using a network provider or choosing one that is out-of-network. If a provider that is out-of-network is chosen, then you will have to pay more. Otherwise your in-network provider coordinates all of your care, including referrals to specialists and hospital stays.

Preferred Provider Network Plan

Like the POS Plan, this plan also offers two levels. In-network and out-of-network. If you choose out-of-network, the plan usually covers 70 percent of the cost of services.

*   *   *   *   *

Like all else in life, there are two sides to everything. The upside is that health maintenance organizations are good for general care and surgeries. The downside is that if you have a serious illness complicated by unknown causes and requiring expensive diagnostic tests, long-term management, or referrals to specialists, then you may have a problem. So what do you do?

1) You should review your health plan carefully, 2) find out what kind of specialists are in the plan, 3) inquire regarding their formal training (there are also books in the reference section of your library which have information on physicians, their place of training, and credentials), 4) do your homework now regarding what's covered, and what isn't covered. If you find you need something that isn't covered — appeal it. If you still don't get satisfaction, then go to the state medical society to complain, and/or to the state insurance department. The

best methodology is to research HMOs and their benefits and enroll in the most comprehensive plan before you develop a complicated illness.

When you enroll in an HMO through work it is for a one-year period, renewable after each year. Suppose you wanted to opt out of it? According to IRS regulations, there are only certain circumstances in which you can change before the end of the year in which you are enrolled:

- If your marital status changes.

- If there is an addition or loss of an eligible dependent.

- If you move out of the service area of the plan.

- If your spouse loses coverage from another plan.

- If there is termination or commencement of your spouse's employment.

What Is the Cost of Enrolling in an HMO if You Don't Have Coverage from Your Employer?

Health maintenance organizations do not usually operate nationwide. They may operate in several states, and rates may vary between organizations. In New York and New Jersey, the Cigna HMO plan costs an individual enrollee $821.36 per month, and the Point of Service Plan costs $1,093.56 per month. In Oxford, the HMO plan is $733.00 per month, and the Personal Freedom Plan is $1,038.38 per month.

When you enroll through your employer, your premiums are much less because it is an employer group plan.

Here are some examples of an employer group plan per-period payroll deduction:

Here's how much your biweekly contribution will be if you elect...

If your annual salary is... And you	elect this coverage level...	PPO Plan	POS Plan	PPN Plan	Blue Choice Prestige HMO	US Healthcare Premier HMO	Oxford HMO
$ 0 -	Single	$ 15.08	$ 10.77	$ 0.00	$ 7.00	$ 9.23	$ 9.23
$40,000	Family	$ 37.69	$ 26.92	$ 0.00	$ 16.00	$ 23.08	$ 23.08
$40,001 -	Single	$ 22.62	$ 16.15	$ 0.00	$ 10.50	$ 13.85	$ 13.85
$60,000	Family	$ 56.54	$ 40.38	$ 0.00	$ 26.25	$ 34.62	$ 34.62
$60,001 -	Single	$ 30.15	$ 21.54	$ 0.00	$ 14.00	$ 18.46	$ 18.46
$80,000	Family	$ 75.38	$ 53.85	$ 0.00	$ 35.00	$ 46.15	$ 46.15
$80,001 -	Single	$ 37.69	$ 26.92	$ 0.00	$ 17.50	$ 23.08	$ 23.08
$100,000	Family	$ 94.23	$ 67.31	$ 0.00	$ 43.75	$ 57.69	$ 57.69
$100,001-	Single	$ 56.54	$ 40.38	$ 0.00	$ 26.25	$ 34.62	$ 34.62
or more	Family	$141.35	$100.96	$ 0.00	$ 65.63	$ 86.54	$ 86.54

There is a book out now that I strongly recommend for you entitled *The Castle Connolly Guide To The ABCs of HMOs — How to Get the Best from Managed Care.* Here are some extracts that are especially pertinent to terminally-ill and other cancer patients:

• *ISSUES AND CONTROVERSY* •

Lifetime Caps

An issue that has attracted little press attention to date, but is a very critical one to all families, is that of yearly or lifetime expenditure caps. Simply translated, this means a limit on the dollar amount an insurance company will be responsible for during a year or during the lifetime of a policy. It applies in both indemnity and managed care situations. While it affects very few people, it can have a devastating impact on those it does affect.

Some insurance policies have limits of $250,000 a year or a million dollars in a lifetime. While these seem to be huge amounts, they can disappear rapidly in today's expensive hi-tech medical environment, where lifesaving miracles occur daily, but often at great expense. This issue was vividly *brought to the attention of our nation by the tragic case of Christopher Reeve, the film star best known for his work as Superman, who became a quadriplegic after a fall from a horse. Despite his wealth, he found himself impoverished in less than two years as the result of his expensive care and limits of his insurance.*

Families should seek insurance plans, managed care or indemnity, without caps or limits.

• *ISSUES AND CONTROVERSY* •

Referrals to Specialists

One of the very sound and fundamental principles of managed care is the reliance on primary care physicians to deliver preventive and basic medical care, and to appropriately utilize referrals to other specialists. It is for this reason that primary care doctors are often referred to as "gatekeepers," a label many resist.

Patients in some HMOs have complained that their primary care doctors have been too slow to refer them to other specialists, when they, the patient, felt they needed the care of another specialist or subspecialist. This issue has been a major point of contention between HMOs and their members. In fact, it has prompted some HMOs to permit patients to see specialists without a referral from a primary care physician. Sometimes these plans are described as "non-gatekeeper" or "HMOs without walls." Their goal is to remove what some consumers believe to be restraints on choice.

The media coverage of the issue of referrals to specialists has been negative for HMOs. A California HMO was fined $500,000 by the state for failing to make medically necessary referrals. The case involved a nine-year-old girl with a rare tumor who was denied access to a specialist with extensive experience in her problem. Fortunately, the surgeon operated, but when the HMO refused to pay not only his bills but the hospital's bill, even though the hospital was part of its network, the child's parents sued.

Some doctors also have expressed concern about this issue, but from a somewhat different perspective. The concern of the doctors, primarily sub-specialists, is that primary care doctors are sometimes reluctant to refer patients because they may incur some financial penalty and are instead treating the patients themselves. These specialists complain that not only are the primary care doctors depriving them of income but they are often offering care or performing techniques for which they are not properly trained.

When you believe you need the care of a specialist, discuss it with your primary care doctor. If he or she will not refer you, and the conversation has not changed your mind, appeal to the medical director of the HMO. If all else fails you may want to pay for a visit to a specialist yourself. If you believe the problem to be serious, it may be worth it! Also, when being referred to a specialist make certain that the physician has the appropriate training and expertise to deal with your problem. If not, appeal to the HMO and, if necessary, demand to be referred to someone who can deal with the problem appropriately.

• *ISSUES AND CONTROVERSY* •

Denial of Care

Perhaps the most frightening issue to consumers, and the one that has attracted major press and political attention, is that of being denied care. There have been some highly visible cases and lawsuits that have attracted tremendous media publicity. These cases are naturals for media exploitation. They involve a sick or dying person and a large company with a million dollars in revenue saying it will not pay for a treatment that may save the person's life. Unfortunately, these cases always have and always will be with us. Indemnity insurers also deny care to people they insure and they do it for the same reason managed care organizations do: In most cases, the care desired is not covered by the insured person's policy. Also, insurance companies of all kinds typically deny reimbursement for care they deem as experimental. They also deny care if they believe it would be ineffective or wasteful. They are often slow — perhaps too slow — to reimburse for new treatments until they are widely accepted. But this is not just a managed care issue; it's an indemnity insurance issue as well.

This issue was vividly dramatized by the case of a California woman who sued her HMO because it denied a bone marrow transplant to combat breast cancer. Some experts claimed the therapy was still unproven. Other experts claimed it would help—perhaps save the woman's life. Some insurers reimburse for the procedure, other do not. Whether effective or not, the question is moot: The woman died after her HMO refused to pay for a bone marrow transplant and her estate was awarded $89.1 million when it sued the HMO!

Reprinted with permission from the Castle Connolly Guide to the ABCs of HMOs — How to Get the Best from Managed Care. *Copyright 1997 by Castle Connolly Medical Ltd., New York, New York 10155.*

Medicare and Medicaid Knock on Managed Care's Door

Medicare and Medicaid are now partners with managed care. They will be fully integrated in the near future. It is interesting and disconcerting that out of financial desperation, Medicare and Medicaid will join a system that they know is not presently acting in its insureds' best interests. Medicare and Medicaid were the "money mills" for the health care industry for many years and now their formerly deep pockets are nearly empty. A report in 1996 projected that the Medicare Hospital Trust Fund (Part A — which provides hospital coverage) would be exhausted in 2001. This is because in the past there were no real restraints in the system. Now, with baby boomers coming of age, the Medicare/Medicaid population will face hardships like no other generation, except those who experienced the Great Depression. There is another problem. As the baby boomers age, there will be fewer workers to contribute to the Medicare fund. In 1965 there were 5.5 working age Americans for every person over 65*.

Clearly, Medicare and Medicaid must be integrated into managed care for financial reasons and service may be severely curtailed as a result. It is estimated that 75 percent of a person's total lifetime health costs will be spent on an end-stage illness. If services are curtailed, this means there will be less care for those who need it most.

The controversy over health care delivery systems is being fueled by complaints from people all over the country. They are telling their horror stories to Congress in an effort to rally support to effect changes in legislation. There is a bill in Congress to overhaul the managed care system. It has the support of both Republicans and Democrats. Key elements include: 1) the right to sue a health plan for decisions resulting in injury or wrongful death, 2) the right to appeal an HMO's decision as to the proper course of treatment for you, 3) the right to access specialists.

Managed Care in the Home

My experience with different managed care organizations has been in the home care division of health care delivery. When I first started working in home care, there were few patients on managed care programs. Most of our patients still had traditional insurance plans. By 1998, most patients were participants in HMOs or other managed care delivery systems. A patient's stay in home care is much shorter today. Years ago a patient's average stay was two months, depending on the diagnosis. Today, it could be several days to several weeks. The exception for a longer stay is when the patient has a wound that needs daily care. There are strict guidelines for keeping a patient on for longer periods than several weeks.

Some managed care organizations are better than others. Some are "cruel," as one supervisor of mine once said. I can

*By 2030 there will be 2.2 working age Americans for every retiree. (*Health Care Almanac*, 1998).

vouch for that. As a supervisor of a team of nurses who stayed mostly in the field seeing patients, I would frequently have to answer the calls from managed care companies and state our case as to why a patient couldn't be discharged from home care. I know of at least one such company that uses social workers as medical case managers. In other words, nonmedical personnel are functioning in the medical arena and making medical judgements and they are not qualified to do so.

Use of social workers as medical case managers at HMOs is not at all uncommon. When you speak to a case manager at a typical HMO, they frequently do not tell you if they are Licensed Practical Nurses, Registered Nurses, or social workers. Now, social workers perform a unique and valuable service to people in the home, as well as in the hospital. But, in my opinion, their scope of practice should be confined to the psychosocial needs of the patient as well as to obtaining resources in the community for the patient.

My role and that of my nurses is to maximize a patient's wellness. The role of the HMO case manager is to minimize the services in the interest of cost-effectiveness. Therefore, my home care team and the HMO are often at odds with each other. It often comes down to who you get on the phone when advocating for patient care. I shouldn't have to go through a litany every time I need a cancer patient's visit-frequency extended. But I do. How can you, the patient, get what you want from managed care? I'll tell you:

- If you are receiving home care services and you are not satisified with the quality of care you are getting, call the nursing supervisor of the agency providing the care and complain. Supervisors must follow-up on complaints.

- If you are not satisfied with the number of visits you are getting as a result of managed care denials, call the same nursing supervisor and call the health department of your state.

- If you are dissatisfied with your HMO or managed care insurance company, disenroll, if you can, but first find out if you can enroll in another plan. If you are a Medicare recipient, you can disenroll at any time and you can do this at your Social Security office or by completing forms from your HMO. Be sure you are enrolled in another plan before you disenroll in your present plan.

- If you need home care continued and your HMO denies visits altogether, call the HMO case manager and bitterly complain. Many insurance case managers fold under pressure. Also, find out the credentials of the person who has issued the denial. If they have no medical background, challenge the denial.

- Appeal to your physician to intercede for you.

- And perhaps most important of all, call your Congressional representative and demand he or she look into your problem — this will bring prompt action, especially today when many HMO reform bills are pending.

The storm over managed care is not likely to blow over any time soon. If you want to get the best care at a price you can afford, you need to be informed. Know the risks and the benefits. If you want more freedom of choice, then choose the out-of-network option. Not everyone is dissatisfied with their HMO. Talk with others about their experiences.

You want to consider these factors:

- Check on the specialists in the plan. What kind of specialists do they have? And what are their credentials? What schools did they go to? What specialty training did they have? Is he or she Board Certified in the specialty area you need?

- What hospitals are affiliated with the plan?

- Check the health plan rules on emergent care. Will it cover emergent care out of state?

- Check the turnover rate of physicians who have left the plan. Are doctors leaving every few months? This will give an idea of physician satisfaction with the plan.

For Your Information

- Major hospitals in the country that specialize in cancer treatments have clinical trials that patients can participate in. The drugs are provided by the drug company sponsoring the clinical tests. Your cost might be for lab tests and doctor's fees.

- The Hill-Burton Program is a federally funded program for people whose income falls within the poverty guidelines. Many hospitals are required to provide a specific amount of free or below-cost health care. A family of four with an income of $16,450 would be eligible for services. (See Appendix for Chapter 2 for further information.)

- The American Association of Retired Persons (AARP) has a booklet entitled "Know Your Managed Care Rights," which has information on enrollment rights, disenrollment rights, "lock in" in HMOs, and your rights to services, etc. (See Appendix for Chapter 2 for information.)

Since managed care HMOs are everywhere, it stands to reason that changes have to be forthcoming as a result of public pressure. Health care will improve for all of us in the future but it is still in our best interest to know all we can about our health care plans before we are faced with a problem. There is power in numbers and when you have a problem, you need to speak up and reach out.

Chapter Three
Through the Forest of Fear

*Receive at last that thou hast in thee something better
and more divine than the things which cause the various
effects, and as it were pull thee by the strings. What is
there now in my mind?*

Marcus Aurelius Antoninus

I used to say half-jokingly to my friends, "I have so many fears, I don't deserve to live." I was afraid of the dark, of spiders, storms, strangers, strange food, strange anything. I was just plain afraid. But saying, "I don't deserve to live?" Perhaps I felt this way because I equated fear with cowardice, and living requires courage. I was young when I said that. And eventually I did conquer most of my fears (although I do have little nightlights in every room and I don't like to be alone during a storm).

Fears are learned at a very early age. We start experiencing fear of strangers after six months of life. Amazingly, infants learn to control their emotional responses to fear by using such behaviors as turning their heads away from the unpleasant towards something that is pleasant, or at least neutral. As adults, we control our fears by doing the same kinds of things — basically avoidance behaviors. But as adults, our fears can be magnified by complex thought processes that can perpetuate and escalate the fear beyond reality.

Fear can be defined as a conscious apprehension of a threat of danger. All fears are valid to the person experiencing them. In the case of someone experiencing a life-threatening illness, fear is brought to the very forefront of consciousness and the threat of danger becomes a reality.

I've thought about this: it would have been easier to get right to the uplifting things you want to hear about, such as meditation, relieving stress, and so on. But I would be doing you a disservice. How can you cope with your fears, stress, and anxiety unless you know where they are coming from and why they are there? It would be like me putting a sterile dressing on a wound without looking at it and cleaning it first. The dressing might make you more comfortable at first but your wound would only fester and become infected. So bear with me here. I know it is difficult for you now, but my intent is to help you change and free you from being dependent in a world that cannot support your dependency. Fear makes us dependent. We have to face that which causes the most distress. Once we face it, we can work through it by identifying it, discussing feelings about it, and giving you the information needed to help resolve it.

In the introduction, I told you that cancer strikes the entire family, and not just the patient. The fear you are experiencing is being felt by every member of the family, including the children. The children sense there is something being kept from them, and many times patients also sense this. The issues may be somewhat different from person to person but the intensity of fear that is felt by each family member is the same. If left unchecked, fear can destroy the best coping mechanisms available — each other's love, companionship, comfort, and support. Therefore, this chapter has relevance for the entire family. It will alleviate the fears that are common to all of you. Communicate your fears to family members in a group setting. The family thus will serve as a support system for each individual member. Now let us examine the pathology of fear.

Fear is differentiated from anxiety in that anxiety results from an *unconscious* feeling of dread or impending danger. Fear is a *consciously* recognized danger or threat. That is why fear can often lead to a complete denial of the threat. For example, you may have discovered a lump in your breast. You deny the threat by rationalizing that "it's just a cyst." Time may pass (sometimes months) before seeing a doctor. Fear also can lead to self-imposed isolation. You may become withdrawn, irritable, or argumentative. This makes the person who is experiencing the fear even more vulnerable because that person is not likely to ask for help. Engaging in this kind of thought-blocking produces a high level of resistance towards others attempting to communicate with you. You might find yourself making curt remarks like "I'm fine" or abruptly changing the subject. Men especially tend to hide their fears because fear is perceived to be unmanly. Men are more susceptible to denial of illness because the alternative is living with their feelings of shame for being fearful. Fear is your worst enemy. It interferes with your ability to live in the "now." And it can seriously affect your ability to deal with the illness.

Of course, I'm not saying you shouldn't have fear. But wishing it away does not make it go away, either. The only way to deal with fear is by recognizing (1) that it's there, (2) why is it there, and (3) what can be done about it. The most effective way to combat fear is with the power of information. We fear most what we do not know. Information will bring the object of your fear into a manageable perspective that is more reality-oriented than imagination-based.

When I have a patient or a family member who is nonverbal and whom I suspect is fearful, I know I have to spend time alone with him or her. I need to reduce external stimuli like noise or other family members talking. I want that person's own reactions without prompting by others. I'll begin by asking, "Tell me, are you experiencing any particular fear? Do you want to talk about it with me?" Sometimes the answer is a nonverbal message like looking down. I don't take that as a "no" answer, I take that as a "help me" message. "I know the doctor told you that you have cancer, and would like to start chemotherapy. What are your feelings about that?" I try my best to get the patient to start verbalizing his or her feelings because I will get a clue as to what the fear is. Then I can go right to the source of the fear and reduce it to the patient's ability to deal with it.

Let's look at some real fears and see if it helps to bring them out in the open.

Fear of Cancer

People fear cancer for many reasons. Years ago, the word cancer was not spoken out loud because it was synonymous

with death.   There were no treatments to speak of that
compare to the treatments and research of today.   Stories
were no doubt handed down from generation to generation
about how grandfather died of cancer.

Today we still fear cancer but we are able to talk about it.
Today there are advanced treatments, research, and hope for
curing it.

Cancer has been around for many, many years.   There are
more than 100 different forms of cancer.   In 1998, there was
an estimate of 1.3 million new cases diagnosed in the United
States alone.   Sixty percent will live five years or longer and
many will be cancer-free and have the same life expectancy as
someone who never had the disease.   There are new advances
in the methods of early detection of cancer which will
continue to improve the treatment and success rates.   There
are more than 8 million cancer survivors alive today in the
United States.   There are also many people who, while being
treated in hospitals, have experienced unexplained recoveries
where they have gone home without any evidence of cancer.
One hospital well-known for its reputation in the care of the
dying has a 4.4 percent rate of unexplained "cures."   Call it
the work of miracles or the work of the will (I call it both), it
happens!

It is very important that you take an aggressive, active role
in defeating this cancer.   That means you need to learn all you
can about the particular form of cancer you have; learn the
treatment options, choices, survival rates.   Your positive
mental attitude plays a major role in defeating the disease or
prolonging life.   Remember, attitude is everything!

Fear of Procedures

Fear of procedures exists because procedures of every kind
are foreign to us.   We don't know what to expect, or if it will
be painful, and we really fear the results of the tests.
Procedures naturally come with their requisite entourage of
strangers in white coats, and tubes or machines we wish were
never invented.   The environment in which these procedures

take place is often cold, stark, and devoid of color and carpeting. We view procedures as an invasion of our body and we fear anything that looks like or feels like a threat of mutilation. When you're sick, even an intravenous line being inserted can be perceived as threatening.

So whether you're having chemotherapy, radiation, surgery, or any of the numerous "procedures," it is natural and normal to be fearful. Ask questions and have a full explanation given to you so you know what to expect. The first time is the worst. By the second time, you're a pro.

Chemotherapy

Chemotherapy is a drug therapy that kills the cancer cells in your body. A patient may be given one drug or a combination of drugs. The drug is given orally, by injection, or by an IV. You should not feel pain while receiving chemotherapy. How long you receive the treatment depends on where the cancer is. You may have a schedule of every day, every week, or once a month, with rest periods in between. Chemotherapy can either cure cancer or prolong life.

Radiation Therapy

Radiation therapy uses high intensity energy aimed at the specific cancer site. Sometimes radioactive elements are used. Radiation therapy is used to shrink tumors by killing cancer cells. Radiation therapy is also very useful in treating cancer pain that occurs in the bone or tissues. It is not painful. The course of treatment depends on the type of cancer and where it is. Radiation is given either externally or internally. With external radiation, the patient visits the treatment facility five days a week for three to eight weeks. A physical examination is performed on the first visit. Then, after the radiation oncologist examines your medical records, he or she will mark the area on your skin that is the site of the treatment. The first treatment begins on your next visit and usually lasts 1-5 minutes.

Internal radiation uses a radioactive substance like iodine, radium, cesium, or phosphorus. Internal radiation may be used in treating cancers of the kidney, head, neck, uterus, thyroid, and prostate. This form of treatment is higher in intensity than the external form and is administered by surgically implanting a high intensity source of radiation. Some implants stay in place for seven days and some are permanent. You will need to be in the hospital usually for one-day surgery for the implant.

Fear of side effects

Hair loss is a side effect of chemotherapy and sometimes of radiation therapy. The emotional impact of losing one's hair is significant because the change in body appearance is relatively sudden — within 2 to 3 weeks of the first treatment. The reason for hair loss is because chemotherapy (all types) is cytotoxic. That is, it not only kills cancer cells, but normal cells as well. It damages and weakens hair follicles, causing hair to break and fall out. Hair loss is usually confined to the scalp, eyebrows, and other facial hair, but can also affect body hair. Hair loss related to chemotherapy is temporary. The hair will begin to grow back 6 to 8 weeks after the treatment has ended. Radiation therapy can also cause hair loss if the therapy is administered to the head. Sometimes the hair loss associated with radiation is permanent.

However, there is new hope on the horizon that in the future, people will no longer have to suffer the trauma of chemotherapy-induced hair loss. A new compound called GW8510, was formulated by the pharmaceutical company, Glaxo Wellcome. This experimental non-toxic compound has shown good results in inhibiting some chemotherapeutic agents from destroying the epithelial cells of hair follicles. Although further testing is needed, and human clinical trials have yet to be conducted, it is only a matter of time before a solution will be found. The important thing to know, is that scientists are working on it now, and millions of dollars in government grants are being poured into the research.

In the meantime, there is help available from the American Cancer Society. The American Cancer Society has a program called "Look Good...Feel Better." It is a community-based, free national service for women and teenage girls who are undergoing cancer treatment. The program provides certified volunteers to teach beauty techniques to patients to improve their self image. Free make-up kits, pamphlets, and videos are provided. The American Cancer Society can also provide a free wig to patients who cannot afford one.

These are just some of the many wonderful services the American Cancer Society provides. They also provide all kinds of information for cancer patients, as well as many supportive services.

Nausea and vomiting are two common side effects of chemotherapy and sometimes of radiation, although not everyone experiences them. Chances are you have already experienced both of these discomforts in the course of your life. We know that nausea and vomiting can be very debilitating. There is a feeling of loss of control and you may be somewhat dependent on others for help. As a result, your functional role within the family may change and necessitate a shift of responsibility to someone else, which perpetuates feelings of helplessness. Your quality of life is threatened and if symptoms are not controlled, prolonged dependence on others may lead to feelings of despair, hopelessness, and suffering.

The incidence of nausea and vomiting varies with age, gender, and the anti-cancer drug being used. It also varies depending on the other medications that you may be taking. Some people even experience nausea and vomiting *before* treatment begins. This is called anticipatory nausea and vomiting, and it occurs as a result of increased anxiety.

I must emphasize that not everyone experiences these side effects. They vary greatly from person to person. In fact, I have had many patients under cancer treatment who did not have a problem with nausea and vomiting at all. Of the people who did have a problem, we quickly controlled it, and many patients did not have recurring symptoms. With some patients I have used antiemetic (anti-nausea) drugs, and with others, I have introduced strictly stress-reducing therapies that required continual management by a social worker in the home.

I have two stories to tell that will illustrate how supportive therapy can make a marked difference in managing these unpleasant side effects. Two of my patients had severe problems with nausea and vomiting. Jane was receiving chemotherapy; James was not. I will talk about James first.

James had been admitted to the hospital on five separate occasions in a five week period for intractable nausea and vomiting. He had lung cancer. His only treatment had been radiation therapy, which does not usually cause these side effects, although it can occur. He was sent home after the fifth hospitalization with an intravenous antiemetic (anti-nausea) medication. His wife had to hook up the intravenous medication several times a day to an IV line that was already in place in his arm. James was experiencing frequent day and night bouts of nausea and vomiting. He wasn't eating or sleeping. He had a great deal of fear surrounding his disease and his wife was having extreme difficulty in managing her own anxieties over his illness and her role change.

I had an idea. I called the medical social worker and asked her to see James 2-3 times a week to work specifically on reducing his stress. I asked her not to discuss his disease with either James or his wife. Margaret, the social worker, spent time with James in his home viewing stress-reducing tapes, and using imagery and relaxation techniques. I called the doctor after two weeks and asked him to start lowering the strength of the anti-nausea medication. James was off the medication in three weeks and the social worker continued on the same course for another three weeks. After six weeks of only working on stress management, James came out of his cycle of fear and anxiety, began taking control, and was able to plan and eat his meals with no further recurrence of nausea and vomiting. I had James on home care for over one year. He never had nausea or vomiting again. Even later, when we had to introduce morphine for pain management, he did not experience any side effects. The social worker made twice weekly visits for approximately two months. James's overall quality of life improved and was maintained during the entire course of his illness. He was never hospitalized again.

Six months later I had a similar patient. Jane couldn't take anything by mouth because of intractable nausea and vomiting. She had completed her chemotherapy but was so debilitated from the side effects that she had to remain bed-bound and was receiving total parenteral nutrition (TPN) intravenously at home. TPN provides all of the nutritional requirements of glucose, fat, protein, minerals, and vitamins that a body needs to maintain adequate nutrition. Of all the patients I have had, Jane was the only one who needed TPN.

Jane was feeling very hopeless and was unable to care for her young children. I was so excited with the success we had with James, I thought, why can't we try this with Jane? I had to call in a different social worker because of Jane's geographic location. I asked Margaret, James's social worker, to conference with another social worker and explain in detail what she had done with James. It seems that six weeks was the magic number. After six weeks of working on stress reduction, coping techniques, relaxation videotapes, imagery, etc., Jane was off TPN, was out of bed, and was eating on her own! Not only that, she became so hopeful and energized, that she went around the neighborhood on long walks with her kids. Like James, she also never had recurring side effects again. What made these two people so special was their ability to overcome and transform in spite of their illness. It is a lesson in hope, courage, and the belief in your own power of will and self-love. All of us have this same power to overcome and transform.

Some side effects may not be psychogenic in origin, that is, coming from the mind. The cause of nausea and vomiting in relation to chemotherapy is currently thought to be the result of the exposure of the chemoreceptor trigger zone (CTZ) in the brain to known mediators of nausea and vomiting —

neurotransmitters such as serotonin, histamine, dopamine, and prostaglandins. So the object in controlling nausea and vomiting during chemotherapy is to inhibit these neurotransmitters with antiemetic drugs. Other causes for nausea and vomiting in the absence of chemotherapy are brain tumors, gastric irritation, ulcers, metabolic changes, and possible side effects of narcotics.

Treatment for side effects is a priority. Years ago, side effects were thought of as a necessary by-product of the treatment and it was assumed that the benefits of the treatments outweighed the side effects. As researchers came to the conclusion that side effects can impact so negatively on one's life, new drugs became available to manage side effects more effectively. I urge you to get the help you need if you are experiencing side effects. Here is some information for you.

Non-Drug Interventions

The side effects of nausea and vomiting can be controlled with non-drug intervention when the symptoms are mild. Check with your doctor. Whatever the cause may be, it is a priority to manage nausea and vomiting because they will interfere with your positive mental attitude and willingness to fight, and they can keep you from eating at a time when your body needs nutrition to build healthy cells and tissues. The following non-drug interventions can be used concurrently with drug interventions:

- Eat small frequent meals during the day, at least 4-6 times a day.

- Avoid fluids with meals. Fluids fill you up at meal time. You want as much nutrition as you can get.

- Avoid fatty foods like fried potatoes or butter, sauces, or spicy foods.

- Prepare small portions of food ahead of time and freeze them.

- Eat foods like skinned chicken (baked, broiled or boiled), angel food cake, fruit, yogurt, toast, oatmeal, clear broths, crackers, rice.

- Ginger ale that has been standing (no gas). Ginger capsules are available over the counter (ask your doctor first); it is a natural anti-nausea spice, and is sometimes used in medicine.

- Do not lie down for two hours after eating.

- Avoid food served at hot temperatures — this may contribute to nausea.

- An ice pack to the back of the neck — 15 minutes on, 15 minutes off — or a cold towel to the forehead helps nausea.

- Take multivitamins with minerals.

Sometimes there is a development of aversion to foods, or loss of taste. Don't eat your favorite foods when you feel you are going to be sick. This may cause an aversion to these favorite foods when you are well enough to eat.

Because you need to maintain nutrition, the doctor may want you to take Ensure, a dietary supplement containing protein and vitamins which comes in the form of a liquid. There are other brands as well. Each contains, on average, 240 calories per 8 ounce glass. It is usually taken three times a day.

Other non-drug interventions include those practices aimed at alleviating stress and anxiety. These include relaxation techniques, imagery, hypnosis, acupuncture, and meditation. Some will be discussed in the following chapter.

Drug Therapy

The "old standby" for nausea and vomiting is a drug called **Compazine.** It has been in use for many years. Compazine can be taken orally, by intramuscular injection, through the rectum, or intravenously. It also comes in sustained release form: 10-15 milligrams every twelve hours. Personally, I have not had much success with Compazine. It controls nausea in some patients but not in all. If non-drug interventions do not help, then you can ask your doctor to try this or other medications.

Another drug used for nausea and vomiting is called **Zofran**. This drug comes in oral solution form and in 4 milligram tablets and also comes in a 32 milligram single-dose injection, tablet, and oral solution. Zofran can also be given by rectum if the pharmacist puts the tablet in a gel cap. The absorption rate by rectum is the same as when it is taken by mouth. It is usually given by rectum because of the problems in swallowing the patients may experience with nausea. It can also be given intravenously. This drug is commonly used in association with chemotherapy. It is usually given in doses of 8 milligrams, 30 minutes before chemotherapy, then every eight hours for two more doses. I have seen the most success with this drug. I usually ask the doctor for 4 to 8 milligrams, three times a day. Some people only need short-range dosing, that is, only for a few days or until their nausea does not return. It is expensive (about $30.00 a pill) but it is well worth the cost.

Reglan is also used as an antiemetic agent and is also given with chemotherapy treatment. It is not advised for persons with a history of breast cancer, bowel obstruction, or seizure disorders. Another drug, **Tigan**, can be given orally, by rectal suppository, or intramuscular injection. Usual dose is 250 milligrams, three times a day. **Kytril** is a new 24-hour drug indicated for the prevention of nausea and vomiting due to cancer chemotherapy with cisplatin, a chemotherapeutic drug. In one study of 52 patients, 62 percent had a complete response of no more than mild nausea for 24 hours when they were given Kytril before their chemotherapy session. An additional 15 percent had only one occasion of vomiting and a more than mild nausea. It is given intravenously for five minutes before chemotherapy. **Torecan** has a usual dosage of

10 milligrams to 30 milligrams, taken as one tablet, one to three times a day. It also comes in injection form and suppository. It is advertised as being as effective as Compazine at half the price.

The cause of your nausea and vomiting may also be a side effect of a medication you are taking, or the result of a chemical imbalance in your body. For example, if you are taking Digoxin (a cardiac medication), it can build up in your body, especially if you have kidney problems. A buildup of Digoxin is toxic. Signs and symptoms of toxicity are loss of appetite, nausea, vomiting, diarrhea, or visual disturbances. If you are taking Digoxin, you need to have regular lab work done to monitor its levels in your blood. If you are being seen by more than one physician, all of them need a current list of all of the medications you are taking.

Fatigue

Patients who receive radiation therapy report fatigue as the most distressing symptom. Patients receiving chemotherapy report fatigue as the second most distressing symptom. (Nausea and vomiting are top on the list with chemotherapy patients.) In patients receiving radiation therapy, fatigue sets in about two weeks after treatment has started. The cause of fatigue is not clear. But there are immunological substances in the body that are secreted after treatment and they are known to cause at least some fatigue. Also, energy is expended during the treatment in attempts by the body to repair damaged cells. And there is less oxygen in the body because red blood cells, which carry oxygen, are damaged during treatment. This leads to shortness of breath on exertion, and fatigue. Depression, anxiety, and loss of appetite are other causes of fatigue.

When a person has fatigue, there is less interest in life's activities. You become listless, you want to sleep, walking is an effort. Everything becomes an effort, even eating. Needless to say, mental outlook is affected negatively, as you can no longer participate in what previously made you happy.

Fatigue is also a result of continually dealing with the stress of having cancer. Life becomes a drag.

Fatigue is a multifaceted problem. There may be many factors causing the fatigue: i.e. nausea, vomiting, loss of appetite, depression, anxiety. We can't just treat fatigue as a one factor problem. We have to look at everything together. So, what can be done? Well, a balance of activity and rest is important. Often, knowing that fatigue is part of the disease and its treatment helps in coping with the effects. You need to talk about fatigue with your nurse, doctor, and family.

Exercise is very important — set up a walking regimen and perhaps swimming. Endorphins are released during exercise. Endorphins are neuropeptides — amino acids in the brain. They act like morphine to suppress pain. They are linked to learning, memory, control of body temperature, sex drive, and other functions. When you exercise, the endorphins that are released give you a sense of well-being.

Fear of Change — Altered Roles

It's natural to be afraid of a new position, because you haven't done it before. Suppose you're the wife and it is your husband who is ill. In your house, he always made all of the financial decisions, paid the bills, etc. In many ways, he was head of the household. Now he isn't feeling well and is relying on you more every day to do the things he did. Not only are you worried about his condition, but you might be thinking, "I can't do this, I've never had to make these decisions, this is too much to handle." It is a lot to handle. It's not easy taking over. Maybe he's well enough to discuss how to manage the finances or other matters. Try to stay calm through this role change. Remember, he is going through a role change too. Now, he may be in a dependent position and you know he's not happy about that.

Life is full of compromise and adjustment. When someone is very ill, there will always be a need for adjustment of roles within the family. It's how you help each other. Make decisions as a family. There needn't be one person "in control." Plan. Make lists of what has to be done. Whether it's paying bills, shopping, doctor appointments, or calls to make. Making a list helps to put your thoughts in order and helps reduce anxiety.

Fear of Loss of Function

We are accustomed to defining ourselves by our functional capabilities. Our self-esteem is measured by how well we function. We self-assess our mental capacity through our ability to remember, analyze, make judgements, and communicate with others. We also define ourselves by how we function physically. We are accustomed to taking care of our own bodies; bathing, dressing, grooming. There are all kinds of life events that can change how we function. When our level of functioning changes, we fear that we will not be the same. And in truth, we're not. But we're not the same in old age as we were in youth, either. We must redefine ourselves when our functional ability changes or we will experience a sense of loss with resultant grief.

Suppose someone has cancer of the colon and now that person has a colostomy. A colostomy is the creation of an artificial anus through the wall of the abdomen where a part of the colon is brought to the surface. The person can no longer have a bowel movement through the rectum, a normal function that makes him or her like everyone else. There is a real loss here in no longer using that part of the body. He or she will no longer feel the urge to "go." Instead, there will be a "movement" through the colon into a bag adhered to the abdomen. It's an adjustment not to be taken lightly by others. There is real grief in any change of bodily function. It takes a great deal of understanding and compassion to realize what that person is going through. It's an adjustment that will take place, but it takes time.

Life can always be enjoyed no matter what level of function you're at. Many people are adjusting to changes in how they function. Those of you who fear loss of function can work through it by knowing what to expect through reading literature, talking to others who have experienced it, or by attending support groups and communicating with your loved ones and health professionals. I want you to come out and live. Don't isolate yourself because of change. *You* may define yourself by your functional loss. I and others define you by your character, sense of humor, personality, insight, wisdom, knowledge, and love!

Altered Body Image

As we define who we are by how we function, we also define ourselves by how we look. Body image is the subjective concept of how you view your body. The psychological awareness of the body begins in very early childhood. The perceptions we have are formed from a myriad of interactions with others. In other words, our body image is the result of memories, responses from others, experiences, and ongoing self-evaluations. If we approve of our body image, we are self-confident, extroverted, and feel at ease in the company of others. If we disapprove of our body image, we feel less powerful, are more apt to feel guilt and shame, and generally have a lowered self-esteem.

Our society has perpetuated the notion that how we look is our greatest asset and youth is to be treasured and sought after at any cost. It stands to reason that we would fear losing what society tells us not to lose: our youth and our looks. Our sense of failure in having a body image that doesn't hold up to the standards set by a narcissistic society is further increased by the actual assault on the body that comes with some forms of cancer and surgeries like mastectomy, colostomy, and head and neck operations, to mention a few.

It requires a good deal of support and counseling to get a person to an acceptable level of comfort in dealing with an alteration in body image. The psychological impact of having a body that has been altered can be profound. There are fears of rejection, lost identity, loss of control over the body, and loss of self-esteem. I can't emphasize enough the importance of support and counseling in coping with changes in body image. There is a risk that feelings of hopelessness and despair may change the course of the disease and that one's ability to fight with both body energy and mental energy may be compromised. We have to prevent a "giving up" attitude at all costs.

So, what are your options? Well, in some cases, like having a colostomy, maybe your only option is learning to live with it. But people do live with colostomies, and very well. It takes time to readjust to a new lifestyle and to redefine one's "self."

In the case of a mastectomy, you can opt for reconstruction. Reconstruction of the breast is done by several methods. The first method, called an autologous tissue transfer, uses part of your abdominal or back muscle to reconstruct the breast. The second method involves using a silicone-filled implant, which because of controversy stemming from problems, is now only available in clinical trials. However, the FDA recently ruled that implants should be made available again as they have not found justification to limit their use.

Reconstruction can be done immediately after a mastectomy or later on. There are over 40,000 breast reconstructions performed yearly. Recent studies indicate a high rate of satisfaction with reconstruction. There are 180,000 women who are diagnosed annually with breast cancer in the United States. Forty percent will have breast reconstruction. Whatever your choice, reconstruction or no reconstruction, it is a fact that many more women are being helped today through research and community support. You need to re-establish control over your body to maintain your body image. This means looking at it and learning to love it even with its imperfections. Once you have gained control, you can restore your image integrity; once you've restored your image integrity, you can live with hope (see appendix for specific organizations for support).

Fear of Death

Most everyone has a fear of death, which is compounded by our society's refusal to look at it. We spend billions of dollars on illusions for maintaining youth. Society's message is clear: don't get old, don't get sick, and definitely — don't die. Because if you do, we'll hide you behind closed doors, whisk you away in the middle of the night, and pretend it never happened. The media teases our fear into virtual reality by portraying death as gruesome and ghoulish. Part of society doesn't want us to look at it, while another part wants to scare us to death before we do die. Don't think these two patterns are without impact. In society's refusal to look at death, we are cloaking the mystery in a shadow of shame and denying help to those who need recognition from their fellow humans.

Death is thought of and feared within many different contexts. The inevitability of death leads us to wonder how we will die. Will it happen in an accident? Will it happen before I get to see my daughter get married? Will it be in a hospital? Will I have pain? Will it be in my sleep? These thoughts can be disconcerting. People who have strong faith seem better able to cope with these concerns.

There is one fear that rises above the rest in relation to death, and that is the fear of extinction. To be, or not to be? We want to believe in immortality and indestructibility. We feel there has to be a purpose for having gone through life, and we would do anything to keep that life going. A natural extension of going through life is the thought of going through death to somewhere else. Whether it be in the form of reincarnation, or as a soul within an ethereal body is anyone's guess.

What distinguishes our thinking on this subject has a great deal to do with our beliefs — our faith. Is faith rescue thinking? No. Faith is a person's truth that comes from his or her knowledge. Socrates said that knowledge is recollections by the soul that has always existed. He infers that the living come from the dead just as the dead come from the living. There is a duality to all things in creation. He suggests a duality in life and death. Eternity is never ending. Duality then is never ending. (We will talk about the views of three great philosophers later on in Chapter Eight.) I believe that there is life beyond death. I do not believe in extinction. There is reason to hope and reason to believe that death has no sting.

How Children View Death

A child's view of death varies according to his or her developmental stage. For instance, a child of 4-5 may see death as reversible, because parents commonly tell their children that the person who died is "sleeping." Children of that age often assume that the deceased will one day wake up. Between the ages of 5 and 10 there is the notion of the boogie man who comes to claim the dead person. It isn't until after ten years of age that the concept of finality is usually grasped.

In contrast, children of all ages who are terminally ill seem to have a sense of their own mortality. They say things like "I know I am going to die." A study by Eugenia Waechter (1972)[13] demonstrates the understanding and fear of death experienced by the terminally ill child. The study included 4 groups of 16 children aged 6-10. It was found that children in the terminal illness group experienced a significantly higher anxiety and fear score than those who did not have a terminal illness, but who were chronically ill, acutely ill, or healthy. The disease was never discussed with any of the terminally ill children by their families or doctors and it was demonstrated that this was a contributing factor to the high anxiety/fear scores of this group. Psychiatrists recommend discussing the illness with the child. Allow children to verbalize their fears, and let them talk by allowing them to answer their own questions, such as, "What do you think heaven is like?"

Terminally ill children do have a keen sense of what is happening. As painful as it is, you need to talk to them. You needn't be blunt about dying, but you do need to allow them to express themselves. When they look for answers to their questions, be truthful without using expressions like "he's sleeping," when referring to a relative, who has died. Give children a sense of hope. What children need most is love and protection. When they are young, they need to feel safe and secure. If their safety and security needs aren't met, they will exhibit greater fear and anxiety. Stay with them during procedures, tests, and treatments. Don't let anyone tell you to leave the room. You have a right to be with your child 24 hours a day if you want.

Curiously, children can be very accepting of death. They often have thoughts of angels as their protectors, as well as thoughts of God. Children also have a lot of support from adults who are outside the family. People pay much more attention to the sick child than to the sick adult.

There is a fascinating story recently told to me by a pediatric oncologist. He said that he had been caring for a young boy who was in the hospital for eight months. The boy never uttered a word to the doctor, which was extremely frustrating for the doctor. Then, in the middle of the night, the nurse on the unit rushed to awaken the doctor, saying the boy wanted to see him. When the doctor approached the bedside, the young boy said he knew what the doctor was trying to do and he thanked him for taking care of him. Two hours later the boy died. The doctor was fighting back tears as he finished the story.

Some children are lucky. I was lucky. I was born with a hole in my heart, making me especially susceptible to infections in that vital organ. One day, I developed a sore throat, a usual childhood ailment. I was five years old and I remember it like it was yesterday. I became delirious. My temperature went up to 106 degrees and I was rushed to the hospital. It was bacterial endocarditis, an infection that, if untreated in time, is 99 percent fatal. The bacteria from the sore throat entered my blood stream and attacked the weakest part of my body — my heart. The treatment was injections of penicillin every four hours 'round the clock. I was terrified of those injections. I screamed every time. My mother was a nurse in the hospital but they wouldn't let her see me except during visiting hours. I was alone with mean nuns and injections. In my mind, I was being tortured.

One day, I was in my crib when the doctor came storming in, scolding the nurse standing next to me. "Don't you know she could die? She is very sick. I don't want her out of bed!"

Dying? I thought, so that's why I feel so bad. Now I wanted to go to the chapel, across the hall from my room. I sneaked out of my bed when the coast was clear. I couldn't wait to talk to God. I had to tell him its alright. This day is so vivid in my mind. I remember how I prayed. My thoughts were very mature. I said it was OK if he wanted me. I believed I would be with angels. That was very comforting to me. Angels, light, and God. I was filled with love. I was sad for my mother and father. But I wasn't frightened. My thought was, God loves me so much he wants me now. I think many children are able to resolve their fear of death through thoughts similar to the ones I experienced. Remember it is important to be there for children so they feel safe and secure.

The fears we all have are not limited to those just presented. Some others include fear of pain, abandonment, losing our loved ones, not achieving our goals, humiliation. So you see, you are dealing with many fears that have a strong impact on your psychological and physical well-being. These fears, while normal, have to be "quieted" by means of establishing positive thoughts and coping behaviors to regain control so you can live a better life. Fear, anxiety, and stress are all different but are related. Remember, anxiety is a state of apprehension which threatens the ego, and comes from the unconscious mind. Fear is a conscious apprehension of a threat of danger. Stress comes from the fears and anxieties we live with. Living with stress can ruin your ability to appreciate life. Now we're going to work on reducing your stress so you can see your world from a different perspective.

Chapter Four
Overcoming Stress

*Think of the country mouse and of the town mouse, and
of the alarm and trepidation of the town mouse...
How easy it is to repel and to wipe away every
impression which is troublesome or unsuitable, and
immediately to be in all tranquility.*

Marcus Aurelius Antoninus

By now, I think you realize just how much you are dealing with, beginning with negative attitudes, abandonment issues, worry over insurance, fears and anxieties. You know also that I understand and appreciate what you are going through. You are under intense stress. I do not underestimate the impact it must have on you, but I also do not underestimate your potential for overcoming these difficulties. I believe in you. You have an enormous capacity to adapt to change. All you need is the awareness of the "anatomy" of stress, as well as the awareness of the stressors that are affecting your body and your mental attitude. You and your family are experiencing the same multivariable conditions of stress.

Remember, in the last chapter, how we went through the Forest of Fear? Remember that I told you that in order to come to terms with fear, you have to understand where the fear is coming from? Well, it's the same with stress. At this point you might be thinking: "Oh no, not again. When is she going to lighten up?" Very soon, dear friends, very soon. You will recognize everything I'll be telling you. By bringing it out to the forefront of your consciousness, you will be better able to cope with that which you now know. There is reassurance in knowing that the stressors you are experiencing are experienced by almost everyone in your situation. You are unique in who you are, but you are not unique in what affects you. Let's see what this stress is all about. Then you can kick it out of your life.

Stress is the non-specific response of the body to any demand made upon it, according to Hans Selye, a leading expert on stress. A stressor is a stress-producing factor, including heat, cold, illness, and psychological pressures, such as failure, loss, and success.

There are good stressors, like getting a new job or feeling excited and happy. There are bad stressors, like illness, infection, fears, anxieties, and self-defeating negative thoughts. When we experience stress (either good or bad), the body reacts. There are complicated mechanisms that go into action to cope with stress. These mechanisms occur at a biological chemical level in your body.

The Anatomy of Stress - The Biochemical Mechanism of Stress

The hypothalamus is a portion of the diencephalon of the brain. It controls and activates the peripheral nervous system, endocrine systems, and many functions of the body, such as temperature, sleep, and appetite. The hypothalamus detects changes in body chemistry and blood pressure. It is also informed of emotional changes via signals from the cerebral cortex (the surface of the cerebral hemispheres — your gray matter). When the hypothalamus senses stress, it sets in motion a series of chain reactions that produce an adaptive response called the General Adaptation Syndrome.

This General Adaptation Syndrome acts through two pathways. The first pathway involves the sympathetic nervous system, which can accelerate the heart rate, constrict blood vessels, and raise blood pressure. This first pathway response is called the alarm reaction.

The second pathway of the General Adaptation Syndrome involves the pituitary gland and the adrenal cortex. This is called the resistance reaction. This resistance reaction lasts for a much longer period of time than the alarm reaction. Basically, during the resistance reaction your body is producing sugar for energy, and is conserving its sodium to allow fluid buildup in your tissue to maintain volume for sustaining blood pressure. You excrete less urine and your fats and carbohydrates are used for energy to sustain the resistance stage of stress.

When you are under stress for long periods of time, these mechanisms have to continue and this places a hardship on your body. This is why people sustain stress-induced illnesses like colitis, ulcers, hypertension, and asthma. Stress, in varying degrees, can also impair judgement and coordination. It can affect your relationships with friends and family due to changes in behavior and maladaptive communication patterns. Stress-related behavior may be exhibited as irritability or anger. Maladaptive communication patterns are those that do not foster communication, such as avoidance, screaming, or using verbal attacks on others.

Look around you. Everyone in the family is experiencing the same stress. The "bad" stress manifests itself in behavior that is counterproductive to achieving emotional stability. They need your help — and you need theirs. All of you are going to have to work together to change so there can be a communal, in-sync effort to manage the collective stress that you all are experiencing. What follows are the medical stressors that affect the entire family. I can help you with these.

Where Your Stress Is Coming From

What strikes me immediately is the predicament you are faced with when the physician explains that you have a serious illness. You are expected to make decisions concerning various treatment options at a time when you are still reeling from the incomprehensible news. You expect your doctor to say which treatment you will be given and when. But that's not the case. You are given a choice of various treatment options and are then asked which course you want to choose. One expert may say one treatment is better while another expert will have an entirely different opinion. Are you capable of making a well-informed decision at this point? No, you are not.

This major source of stress can be managed by taking the following steps:

- I suggest you go to the library and look up an article from *USA Today*, dated June 22, 1998. The article will give you an in-depth view of the problem of deciding on a cancer treatment. It is entitled *"After Cancer: Therapy Choices Boggle the Mind,"* and is written by Tim Friend.

- Next, I recommend that you call your local Cancer Society and request information of every kind on the type of cancer you have and choices of treatment, with expected outcomes.

- Get the opinion of several experts in the field — at least two.

- Have a family member or friend do some computer research on the subject.

- Find out as much as you can before making a decision. Time is of the essence, so make it your priority.

- The more information you have, the more you will be able to cope with the stress of having to make that decision.

The apparent inattentiveness of other people can not only be an irritant, but a surprisingly significant stressor, as well. How many times have you been to a doctor's office expecting polite, courteous attention from the receptionist or assistant? A smile may be all you are looking for, or a warm pat on the shoulder for reassurance. What you often encounter is a brisk person who is only interested in making sure the bill will be paid. But keep in mind that you are often dealing with someone from an age group with no concept of illness or mortality: they truly believe it will not happen to them, therefore, it is impossible for them to empathize.

- Do not take it personally.

- If poor treatment of a loved one bothers you, you could say something like, "My mother is very ill and she is scared. I would appreciate a gentle, kind manner from you when you speak to her." say this when your mother isn't present.

- Mention your concerns to the doctor. Often, the doctor is not aware of how the office staff communicates with the patients. Your doctor will welcome your comments.

A major stressor occurs when the constraints of work conflict with your desire to stay home to care for your loved one. You may need the income to support the household budget. Most households now need a two-person income. And what if there are young children involved who can't be cared for by mommy because she is ill?

- There is the Family and Medical Leave Act of 1993, which requires employers of fifty or more people to provide unpaid leave for up to twelve weeks to their employees who need to care for a family member or, for their own serious condition. The employer still has to provide medical coverage and ensure the employee of a comparable job upon return to work.

- Consider a private-hire situation where you could employ a person with notable references to care for the children and/or the person who is ill. You might also want to consider hiring a live-in aide. Contact your community home health agency. There is a listing in your local telephone book under "health." Licensed home health agencies have live-in and shift help on staff. While it is an adjustment in the beginning, the value of having another person in the home who can share the responsibilities of care and home maintenance is immeasurable. It can greatly reduce the burden of stress.

- Consider taking out a bank loan to cover costs of a home health aide. Usually, people remain pretty self-sufficient and ambulatory for a long time during a major illness.

There may be a need of only several weeks to several months of home help.

- Consider asking a relative to help.

The stress of financial worries can be a particularly heavy load. Everything comes at once: the doctor bills, hospital bills, treatment bills, medication costs, etc. There is some help for you out there, but not total relief.

- If you are not on home care services through the community or through the hospital, contact a Certified Home Health Agency in your community. Ask for one or two visits from a social worker. You will have to pay out-of-pocket for this (home care will be discussed in the following chapter). A social worker will not only tell you what you are entitled to, but will help you with the forms and the paperwork needed.

- If your loved one is terminally ill, you can apply for Social Security Disability payments, regardless of his or her age. Contact your nearest Social Security office. They also may provide survivor benefits for you and your children. Inquire.

- Regarding medications: you may be entitled to receive several months' supply of medications at no cost. The usual income for eligibility is up to $25,000 or $40,000, depending on different criteria. See the appendix at the back of this book for a partial medications list and the corresponding manufacturer. You can send for the complete list by writing to the United States Senate, Special Committee on Aging, Washington, DC 20510-6400. Ask for the Guide to Low Income Medication Assistance Programs. This guide is a 44-page booklet.

The Stress of Feeling Inadequate in Providing Care

There is always the feeling of being scared and inadequate when trying something for the first time. Remember — your life is made up of hundreds of first-time tasks, tasks that you have mastered and are comfortable with now. Providing care for a loved one is very special. This is your private time together, a time to bond and a time to grow. You, as the family member, are the most important resource your loved one has. With practice, inadequacy becomes proficiency. If your loved one needs help with colostomy care, foley care, injections, etc, you can most certainly learn what you need to do and feel comfortable with it. Once you learn a task, the stress goes away. Where you once felt inadequate, you will feel in control. You will never be expected to do anything until you are taught first. Your nurse will train you and you will continue to have the nurse's support until you are comfortable with doing a procedure.

You may ask, "Why do I have to learn?" It has to do with you taking responsibility for your loved one. It also has to do with health insurance. If the cost of nursing care is paid for by insurance, whether it be Medicare or an HMO, they expect the family members to learn certain procedures and provide physical care. Years ago, nurses would take charge of doing this care in the hospital. However, due to early discharges from the hospital (demanded by managed care), patients are being sent home with a multitude of care needs. Now it's up to the family to carry on these tasks, but only with the help of a nurse who teaches the procedure and then monitors the patient's progress on an intermittent basis. Some procedures can only be done by a nurse and the family is not expected to learn these. I will explain, in the next chapter, what it is that you will need to know. Your feelings of inadequacy will soon give way to feelings of pride and strength.

At this point, I would like you to think about what you have learned from the beginning of this book, starting with

Chapter One. You now know about attitudes, insurance, fears, and stress, and how these will affect the entire family. Now I want you to come with me on a visit to a patient and his family. What you will see is not a unique situation. In fact, it is the rule, rather than the exception, a reality that many families experience.

When I first walk into a patient's home, everything is initially quiet. I introduce myself. Within five minutes, someone invariably makes a comment that sets the other one "off." Arguing ensues back and forth. Things get slammed down on the table, voices rise, and screaming or yelling follows. One person may leave the room in a huff while continuing to argue from a distance, (usually from the kitchen). Drawers slam, dishes clink loudly, epithets fly back and forth like arrows intended to strike at the heart. Does this sound familiar to you?

Meanwhile, I'm just sitting on the couch silently watching... and learning. I'm gathering my data. I believe they want me to see this, otherwise they would have abruptly stopped. They are asking for help — without asking. Who's talking? Who has started the argument? What is the patient doing in response to this commotion? Is the patient the cause of the commotion? I have noticed the breakfast in front of the patient — untouched. What time is it?, I ask myself. I look at my watch. It's noon. What are they saying to each other? Is the patient fighting back or is he passive? Who is the person that just came in, looked around, and then went upstairs? Does the patient look at me or is his head down? I wait as long as it takes. I don't try to interrupt this dynamic situation because I'm learning about my patient's needs and the needs of the family.

After the situation calms down, I usually have enough information. My information tells me, first off, that this family needs help. Secondly, I know who is in control — the wife. She may not be in control of her behavior, but she is the one who is making the decisions, and she seems uncomfortable with this. Thirdly, I know by my patient's response of holding his head down and closing his eyes that he is only reacting when forced to. He is either passive, passive aggressive, and/or depressed. (I would explore this further on later visits.)

This information is very important to me at this time. My goal is to try to change the behavioral posture of everyone in the family because if I don't, there will be increased physical and emotional pain, increased stress, and a total inability to cope on the part of all concerned. We will come back to this family in a little while.

Not every family is like this, but I have encountered many — probably two thirds of my cases were just as I described. Do you think they are ready for deep breathing exercises? No way. It won't work because their stress level is too high. They're playing psychological games with each other — maybe not consciously — and as long as that is going on, they cannot progress to a better level of functioning. I know intuitively that unless the family understands why they are behaving like that, they won't be able to change the pattern. I take one step at a time. First, I have to make sure my patient is stable physically. I can't work on stress reduction until I know that there are no physical problems at the time. Then I look more closely at how stress is affecting the patient and family and I try to talk to them about it.

This can be a tricky process, but it is very important. Unfortunately, people who are under extreme stress cannot take in too much information. Yet they need information in order to reduce the stress. Attention spans are short and people under stress fatigue easily. This is a major problem because some patients do not have the luxury of time to learn all they have to know in order to accomplish the goals of 1) finding themselves, 2) coming to terms with mortality, 3) living with quality, 4) having freedom from pain, 5) being cared for and/or dying with dignity.

I have found that relieving stress will help accomplish all five goals. Think about it. You won't be able to find yourself if you're lost amidst a sea of confusion and stress. You won't come to terms with mortality because you can't see beyond the stress. You won't live with quality because stress negates quality. You will have more pain because stress enhances pain. You may not have quality care at home or die with dignity, because stress can interfere with a caregiver's ability to give care. What you all need to know is that unless "bad" stress is greatly reduced, the goals we have set together cannot be accomplished.

Sometimes within that first week of seeing the patient, I want to make a second visit for the purpose of talking with everyone in the family. I ask if they could all be present for my next visit. At that next visit, when we're all sitting down, I would talk about the situation I found on my first visit. It might go something like this: (John is the patient; Mary is his wife).

Me: I know you are under a lot of stress. [Then I tell them how stress works on the body and depletes the energy needed to help the body.] Do you mind if we talk about the behaviors I saw? [I must always get their permission to enter this private area.] These behaviors are very common among patients and families who are going through a traumatic experience. My intent is to help you through this difficult time. It can make such a difference if we look at why this happens. Can we talk about it?

Mary: OK, fine [she looks at John].

John: OK, go ahead.

George: Sure.
(son)

Me: What I saw was a pattern of arguing, a back and forth match that escalated into screaming and banging things. Remember? Mary, you became so upset that you left the room and continued to yell. John, you were saying things too, but you were more passive. And George, when you came in, you went right upstairs. Can you tell me what started it?

Mary: John wouldn't eat. He never eats.

John: You nag me all the time.

Me: John, why can't you eat?

John: I feel nauseous. I can't taste anything.

Me: Are you nauseous all the time or some of the time? Can you tell me when this happens?

John: It comes and goes, but I have no appetite.

Me: John, you may be taking medications that have a side effect of nausea. I know this is distressing to you but we will work on taking care of that. Your stress may be giving you nausea, also. [At this point I would suggest foods to eat and foods to avoid.] I want you to tell me on a scale of 0-10, with 10 being the most, what number is your nausea?

John: A five. [I now know that John's nausea is preventing him from having a normal day. It's too high. I will have to call the doctor and ask for an antiemetic medication.]

Me: Mary, do you feel like you have a lot of stress?

Mary: My God, yes! I can't do this by myself. I don't know what he needs. I have to do everything now.

Me: What is it that is overwhelming you?

Mary: I have to take him to the doctor, pick up his medications, pay the bills, cook the meals, take care of the house.

Me: George, can you help with any of these responsibilities?

George: Sure, but she doesn't ask me!

Me: George, why don't you ask her what she would like
        you to do. Maybe you can help her by driving your
        dad to the doctor.

        Now I'm going to come right out and ask you — all of
        you — what are you most afraid of? You may have
        questions that perhaps I can answer. You are not
        alone in this. The more we talk about it, the more it
        will help. John, are you afraid of anything?

John: I'm afraid of losing my family. [John starts to cry.
        This is very good because we have opened the gates
        for communication and he is "allowed" now to express
        his feelings to his family.]

Me: John, remember one thing first. There is always
        hope. The second thing is that your family is here
        with you. They will continue to be here with you.
        Your family loves you very much. I would like to have
        a social worker come here and talk to all of you. A
        social worker can help in coping with stress. She can
        also help with getting any financial entitlements if
        you have financial needs. John, there is a lot of help
        available to you and your family. We'll work on one
        thing at a time, alright?

        Do you have any other concerns, like pain, or questions
        regarding your illness?

John: Will I have a lot of pain?

Me: No, John you won't. If you start having pain, I need
        to know about it right away. It's possible to be lucid,
        pain-free, and as alert as you are now. But you have

to tell me about any pain if it should occur. What I do is ask you to rate your pain on a 0-10 scale with 10 being the most severe pain. You give me a number and that's how we keep track of it. I will post a flow sheet in the house that will have the numbers you give me. The pain medication will then be given to keep you between a zero and level two. You should not worry about addiction occurring. It rarely happens. If there are side effects like nausea or feeling like you want to sleep all the time, we can handle that too. OK? Does that make you feel better, knowing about what we would do?

John: Yes.

Me: Good. Mary, is there anything you are afraid of?

Mary: I don't know what to expect. Not knowing scares me.

Me: Well John still has a lot of living to do. And so do you. All of you have a lot of living to do. I want you to enjoy the time you have. I want you to try and make it special. Once we get John's nausea under control, then you can start living in the love of each other. Right now, he's not up to talking too much or taking part in any activity because of the nausea. I hope to have that under control within a day. As far as what to expect, can you tell me more about what you mean?

Mary: What will I need here for him?

Me: You may not need anything. But the most you will see in your home is a hospital bed if John becomes too weak and needs someone to care for him. He may need oxygen if he has shortness of breath. And if he should develop severe pain, then there may be an intravenous line put in. But you needn't worry about that now. See? John, you're doing very well.

You don't have to have these things. It is all your decision. Sometimes knowing what might be in the home can relieve your anxiety. I can promise you this: John will remain comfortable. Did I answer your question?

Mary: Yes.

Me: Mary, when John doesn't eat, try not to take it personally. If he doesn't eat, it's because he can't eat, right John?

John: Right.

Me: I'm going to call the doctor for a medication to help the nausea. I'll ask the pharmacist to deliver it so you don't have to go out. I will call you tomorrow to see if it has helped. Is there anything else you want to tell me? George, why don't you say what is on your mind?

George: I just let them handle it. I'm not around much, you know, I work.

Me: I think all of you need to be together as much as possible. And George, your mom and dad need you now, even if it's just to talk. I would like the three of you to sit down like this and just talk like we have. You don't need another person like me, unless you want me here. I think it helps to talk and what will help more is that you do it at least twice a week.

George, we all have one life. We can't change things from the past. We can change some of the future. My point is that I don't want anyone to have regrets. Do you know what I mean? If anyone has anything to say, then now is the time to say it. I don't mean this minute, but you should tell each other how you feel.

Love is a powerful thing. It heals, it comforts, and it sustains us. If you want to tell your father you love him, please tell him. And John — if you want to tell your son you love him, please tell him. All of you need to hear it said. Don't assume they know. Everyone needs to be told. OK?

Another thing: stress can affect our behavior as well as our bodies and health, as I explained before. The arguing is a result of being stressed. Unkind words being said to each other is a result of being stressed. When this happens, I want you to try and stop for a minute and remember that stress is causing the situation. All you have to say is, "Alright, let's talk about why we're fighting. What is it that is really on your mind?"

I have given you a typical composite family example, although the situation is not fictitious. I have seen this situation many times with families from diverse economic levels. Whether they are well-to-do or poor, they manifest stress in the same ways.

When I talk about the need to change, I am referring to behaviors. You need to change your behavior. If you argue frequently with someone in the family, you need to stop that. If you are quiet and are suffering in silence, you need to talk. If you avoid situations by running away, you need to come back home and work it out. If you don't work things out now, you will be stopped in your tracks later — maybe years later. Regret lingers in your heart like an anchor. As difficult as it is for you now, pull that anchor up so as not to be encumbered by it for the rest of your life.

What about the other families, the ones that are different from the stressed family I have just described? Well, they may be different in several ways. The first thing I notice when I make a visit to a "different" family is that their home is in order, literally. They are organized. The other families have their lives out on the dining room table, and there is confusion and problems in remembering things and locating information they need. The organized family has a place for everything. They think in an organized manner. They are much less stressed.

Another way they are different is in their relationships with each other. There is a strong family bond of mutual support and interactive communication; opinions of others are respected and decisions are mutually agreed upon. They also appear to have a strong faith in God. This allows them to share their burden with Him. They trust in divine intervention, which gives them their strength to persevere in spite of counter influences.

Can you learn to cope like this? Yes, you can. You can begin by getting organized. This will help you organize the way in which you think. Make lists of things you need to do and number the items in priority sequence.

In addition, we're going to use the following adaptive behaviors to further control stress, especially for the cancer patient:

- **Focus on positive energies** like hobbies, recreation, and social activities. Make a list of everything positive you like to do. For example: looking at family pictures, viewing videos, old movies, comedies, writing poetry, reading a novel, seeing friends, taking a walk.

- **Start doing** your favorite things from your list.

- **Talk your problems out** — talking about what is on your mind will reduce your stress. Don't be afraid that you will worry your spouse or family. They will be relieved that you brought it up.

- **Take control** — start taking control of your environment by making small decisions on your own, like planning your meals.

- **Voice your opinions** — tell your family what it is you want from them. Go ahead and say it. "George I need your help. I think you should help your mother by doing the checkbook. It's difficult for her and I'm not feeling well enough to do it. Will you do that for us?"

- **Think positive thoughts** — think of yourself doing the things you like to do. Close your eyes and imagine you are strong, energetic, and happy. Think of happy times in the past and project happiness for the day and for tomorrow.

- **Bring love back into your life** — say "I love you" often to everyone in the family. Hold the hand of your spouse while watching TV. Kiss each other, hug each other. Love is a positive energy. Do all you can to fill your world with love, because love brings happiness, hope, safety, and security.

Using Imagery to Control Stress

Imagery is a therapeutic approach to decrease stress by using the imagination to create a positive, pleasant environment. The goal is to replace negative thoughts with positive thoughts of peace and healing. It requires concentration to create images. It also requires a distraction-free setting.

I was amazed the first time I used imagery. I didn't know how to start or what to do, but the situation I was in required fast thinking and a "wing it" approach. Here is how it happened:

Megan

I was at the home of my patient. She was young, beautiful, and in the last stage of life. The intravenous therapy nurse was already there and had attempted to start an IV several times without success. Megan's veins were poor. She was constantly retching and spitting up, because of an abdominal obstruction. I stood there feeling helpless. Her husband looked at me with such a pained expression that I had to think of something.

We were in the living room and Megan was sitting in her favorite chair. Her face grimaced every time the needle was inserted and pulled out again. Her retching and spitting up continued all the while. I grabbed a chair and sat in front of her, very close. I asked the IV nurse to stop a minute and wait for my signal. I had no idea of what I was going to do next. I told them I hadn't done this before and to just bear with me, that it might take some time. I took hold of Megan's left hand. The IV nurse was kneeling on the floor with her equipment ready. I asked Megan to close her eyes and breathe slowly in through her nose. I told her she was going on a picnic. This is how I continued: "Megan, I want you to imagine yourself at a beautiful park. It's a summer day. The sun is warm on your face. The grass is such a beautiful emerald green. Feel the grass, Meg. It's so soft. You can see the pond right next to you. There's a beautiful white swan gently gliding by. She's beautiful. There's peace all around and the soft breeze on your face is comforting. There's a huge weeping willow tree there hanging over the pond. Your husband is here with you, holding your hand."

I noticed that shortly after I had begun, she stopped retching. I continued speaking in a low, soft voice while repeating the different images and sensations. Ten minutes had passed. She had fallen asleep and I nodded for the IV nurse to try again. She got a vein on the first try and Megan was still asleep when the IV nurse finished. I wanted to let her continue on her picnic with her husband. I whispered that I'd be back later. As I walked out of her home, with tears streaming down my face, I said, "Thank you God."

You can do this for yourself. Begin by lying in a comfortable position. Close your eyes and breathe slowly, inhaling through your nose and exhaling through your mouth. Relax all of your muscles. Think: in 2... 3... 4... out 2... 3... 4. Imagine tension leaving your body as you breathe in 2... 3... 4... out 2... 3... 4. Listen to the sound of your breathing. Think, "I am deeply relaxed." Now let your thoughts wander to a place of peace and tranquility. It may be in a forest with a waterfall, or on a beach with blue water. Birds could be singing. Let lush plants, cool breezes, and water fill your senses. Make your special place beautiful. When you are ready to return, fade your images gently and think of breathing again. In 2... 3... 4, out 2... 3... 4. When you are ready, open your eyes slowly and sit or lie relaxed for a while. Try to remember your "place of peace" and enhance it every time you go back to it.

Relaxing Your Muscles

Do you notice how tension accumulates in your muscles? Your neck can be tense or your shoulders. Doing progressive relaxation techniques can relieve some of that tension caused by stress. Here's how:

- Sit in a comfortable chair. First start with your upper body. Tense all of your facial muscles, including your forehead. Hold the tension for five seconds and release. Now make your facial muscles feel limp. Keep the limp position for ten seconds.

- Next, tense your arm tight. Hold it. Hold it. Then release. Let your arms hang down at your side limp. Feel the pleasure of relaxation.

- Do the same with your buttocks, then upper legs and lower legs and feet.

Take deep breaths like before by inhaling through your nose and exhaling through your mouth. Try to stay relaxed for fifteen minutes.

Massage

Massage can be used to relieve stress. It is very relaxing and involves stroking, kneading, pressing, and squeezing the skin. Massage should not be used, however, if the person has a blood clot, an unstable spine, or an infection of any kind.

Anyone can give a massage and it is very soothing emotionally, as well as, being a stress reducer. Massage gives a person a feeling of well-being because touch is an important way of communicating this feeling.

Back Massage

Begin by warming a bottle of lotion in warm water. A non-oily preparation is best. Have the person lie down on the bed on his or her stomach. It helps to have the room darkened. Apply the warmed lotion to the skin of the back. Begin at the bottom, using the pads of your fingers on either side of the spine, and work your fingers in a circular motion while moving up the sides of the spine. When you get to the top of the shoulders, bring your hands down the sides. Then you can use the heel of your hands to repeat these motions. You can use the same steps for the legs and arms. Always start at the bottom, working up and out.

Getting a Good Night's Sleep

If you are stressed, you are most likely not getting a good night's sleep. How you sleep at night affects the quality of your next day. A restful sleep can reduce your stress.

- Try to stay awake during the day. If you need a nap, take a short one. Use an alarm clock and set the time for one hour.

- Avoid caffeine, chocolate, and colas at night.

- Exercise during the day.

- Avoid drinking fluids after 7 P.M. (this may help in fewer trips to the bathroom).

- Eat a light snack before going to bed.

- Use your relaxation techniques before closing your eyes.

- Don't go to bed angry.

You can also try taking a warm bath or shower before going to bed. A relaxing back massage will help, too. Read about something you don't care to read about; boredom will put you in a restful slumber! If you still encounter difficulty in getting a good night's sleep, ask your doctor for help. There is also help available from Searle Pharmaceutical, which has an audiotape and booklet about *"Easy Steps to Help You Sleep"*. Call 1-800-9 Shut-eye.

Using Humor to Send Stress Away

Laughter, they say, is the best medicine. I think they are right. Countless people have used humor to control pain, heal broken bones, relieve depression, and fight infection, among other things. Humor inspires hope, and where there is hope, there is the will to live.

Living with cancer is no laughing matter. You may be thinking, "Who can possibly laugh at a time like this?" A man by the name of Norman Cousins, who was editor of the *Saturday Review* and a best-selling author, used laughter to combat a life-threatening form of arthritis. After spending some time in the hospital, he convinced his doctor to allow him to set himself up in a hotel.

Cousins implemented a program of daily viewing of funny movies that were sure to produce belly laughs. The doctor took sedimentation rates before, as well as hours after the laughing episodes. (A sedimentation rate is the rate at which red blood cells settle in a tube of unclotted blood. When there is inflamation of the tissue in the body, the sedimentation rate will be high.)

What they found was that the sedimentation rates dropped after each laughter treatment. They continued to drop as the testing went on. What this means is that the laughter seemed to have a beneficial physiological effect on his body. There is definitely a mind-body connection. Laughter also relieved his pain for several hours at a time. Interestingly enough, Cousins made a remarkable recovery from his illness. Laughter is a "good" stressor; and like a "bad" stressor, sets off the same biological mechanisms I spoke about earlier, including the release of endorphins, which are ten times more potent than morphine in blocking pain.

This is just one example of how laughter can relieve stress, reduce inflamation, and relieve pain. So get out your Seinfeld, Three Stooges, or Marx Brothers videos, and your joke books and funny novels. Laughter is a serious medicine, a medicine you can take with pleasure.

*   *   *   *   *

There will always be one kind of stress or another to contend with. The good stress I spoke about can motivate you into action, while the bad stress can drive you into despair. Only you can change how stress affects you. By overcoming stress, you will be free to live your days with quality. You will be able to draw nearer to those you love, and enjoy the things in life that are meaningful to you. Practice the relaxation techniques. Make them part of your everyday routine. Learn about yourself. Look within. You hold the answers to your own questions. Love yourself; Love of self can hold negativity at bay. Allow only positive thinking into your life. You are strong with the will to live. Use that strength to keep yourself in your place of calm — stay there and you will see a change.

Chapter Five

Home Is Where the Heart Is

When thou wishest to delight thyself, think of the virtues of those who live with thee; for instance, the activity of one, and the modesty of another, and the liberality of a third, and some other good quality of a fourth…wherefore we must keep them before us

Marcus Aurelius Antoninus

Home is where your heart is. Home...what do you think of when you think of home? If I asked you now to close your eyes and think of home, what would you see? You would see what has made you who you are today. You would see your entire life lived within the bosom of your family. Perhaps you would see yourself as a child growing up with your mother and father. If you have brothers and sisters, you would remember how their pranks caused you to scheme for revenge in a world of make-believe. Remember how you would rush out to play and then run faster than the wind to get home? Home is a safe place where you have grown up and tested the uncertain and fearsome world from a distance.

Your values were born there, as were your thoughts for achieving your seemingly impossible dreams. Home has given you the courage to reach out and touch the tips of possibilities. It is a place where we all feel secure because of the acceptance of who we are. There is no vying for power or position there. Our home gives us the prerogative of keeping the rest of humanity at the dividing line between chaos and peace — the door. We are free, loved, honored, respected, and enjoyed there. This is why we want to be cared for at home when we are ill.

As a cancer patient, there will be times when it is necessary to have the intervention of medical professionals to oversee and manage your care. However, hospitalizations are not always necessary. Most care that has traditionally been given in a hospital is now given in the patient's own home.

Being cared for at home has special significance and purpose. Your family members are there with you or can visit any time. You have the opportunity to maintain your privacy and sense of control. Your nutritional status will most likely remain the same or improve because you will continue to eat your favorite foods, when you want them and prepared the way you like. A home environment is always best for maintaining nutrition, comfort, and rest.

Most importantly, you are less likely to be at risk for infection when you're at home. Hospital-acquired infections are common. Two million hospital-acquired infections are reported each year (*USA Today, 8/26/99*). In a hospital you are exposed to viruses and bacteria in the air, as well as surface contaminants. There are bacteria on doorknobs, bed rails, privacy curtains, and a host of other sources - even on the hands of your caregivers. In short, you are exposed to many potential transmitters of infections. Of course, your own home also has bacteria. The difference is that your home is an environment you have lived in and you have acquired a resistance to its microorganisms.

If you are receiving chemotherapy, radiation therapy, or other cancer-related treatments, there is an added risk for infection related to the effects of the treatments (decreased white cells, decreased red cells, tissue damage, inflamation, decreased immune response, etc.). If you are receiving cancer treatment, you are far better off being cared for at home rather than being exposed to infectious organisms, many of which are now commonly resistant to antibiotics.

There are many situations that would entitle you to receive home care. A more detailed description of the criteria follows later in this chapter. In essence, if you are homebound or have recently been a hospital patient and have a "skilled need" for a nurse or therapist, then you would qualify for home care. Almost anything that is done in the hospital — with the exceptions of surgery, invasive procedures, blood transfusions, and radiation therapy — can be done in the home.

You don't have to be bed-ridden or dying to receive home care. Very often a cancer patient just needs short-term care to get through the rough times of symptom management.

Once the patient is stable and physically able to return to his or her prior level of functioning, then he or she would be discharged from home care in the same manner that a patient would be discharged from the hospital.

Because this book is for all cancer patients and their family members, it is necessary to address home care for the terminally ill cancer patient as well. The only difference is that care for the terminally ill would be more comprehensive in nature and would continue as long as the patient needed it.

Why We Want to Die at Home, with Dignity

Just what does it mean to die with dignity? We all have our own definition of that, and probably dignity means different things to different people. I can only give you my perspective on dying with dignity. I do know that everyone wants to keep their dignity intact especially when approaching death. Although it may never be concretely discussed, the desire for dignity seems to be communicated by patients in nonverbal ways, such as when they respond in a positive manner when they are being cared for with love. You just know when they are content.

Death in itself is not dignified. The fact that death is inevitable doesn't mean it is dignified or even acceptable. The struggle for life at the end bears witness to our natural resistance to letting go. If death is not dignified, then how does one die with dignity?

To me, dying with dignity means sparing me the humiliation of crying out in pain, writhing in bed, and having to beg for help from those who can't or won't help. It means sparing me from the routine of loud hospital noises, indifference, closed doors, and unwelcome remarks from strangers who cross the dividing line between chaos and peace, a line now drawn at the edge of a hospital bed.

Spare me from prying strangers who are merely satisfying their curiosity, and not showing concern. Spare me from those who would snap the covers away from me to give me a cold bath with cold hands. Spare me the indignity of dying alone without the hands of the ones who know and love me. Spare me the indignity of dying in a place where no one knows my name. Dying with dignity is to die at home, where you are loved, and cared for with love. It is a place where you can die where you have lived. Home is where your heart is. Home is where your dignity is. Dying with dignity is dying at home.

It is very hard for some families to have a loved one dying at home. They are frightened and unsure of whether it is the right thing to do. If you ask your loved one who is dying what he or she wants, the answer might be, "you should send me to the hospital." He or she is probably saying that to avoid being a burden to you. Believe me, no one wants to go to the hospital. Think of what you would want for yourself. Think about it. Do you want to die in a hospital? If you had a choice — what would it be? I would venture to say that you, too, would want to die at home where you would be surrounded by your things: your pillow, your special blanket, your room. It's safe and secure. Your memories are close by. Your pets can comfort you. You would see the trees and birds through your window. These things matter.

What you want for yourself, you should want for a loved one. This is your final, and perhaps greatest gift to your loved one. It is a gift of tremendous value that requires personal sacrifice. Yes, you will be stressed, hurt, and sorrowful. It takes courage to watch someone you love die. It would take courage for someone you love to watch you die. But, it will bring you closer together. And yes, it's going to take time out of your life. But it is time, which hopefully you will have a lot of in your life. Time is something your loved one doesn't have.

Sometimes families change their minds. In the beginning, they may have all good intentions. No one can be judged for the decisions made. Some people just can't handle caring for the dying. Here is one good example of this:

Ralph

Ralph was a patient of mine. His fate was like that of others I have seen. He was in his seventies, and had lived alone in an apartment some distance from his daughter. After Ralph was diagnosed with terminal cancer, his daughter insisted that he come live with her and her husband. Ralph was reluctant to leave his home of forty years and to appease him, the daughter said it would be temporary. Ralph's condition was frail but he was maintained on home care for about one year. He had intermittent bouts of nausea and vomiting, which were quickly brought under control.

The daughter had great difficulty in coping with any change whatsoever in his condition. This necessitated the need for a social worker to work with Ralph and the family for counseling and coping techniques. Ralph was sweet, and gentle, and he never wanted to be a bother to anyone. He always apologized for any inconvenience caused by his not feeling well.

There were two occurrences that dramatically changed circumstances for Ralph. After about a year of living with his daughter, Ralph was told that she had to let his apartment go and his furniture was being moved to her home. Less than two weeks later, he had developed diarrhea and had "made a mess" on her rug. The daughter made arrangements for him to be transferred to a nursing facility the next day. There was nothing either I or the social worker could do to change her mind.

Ralph accepted this with complacency. The only thing I could do was to assure him that he would be well taken care of. I had been to the facility before, and I knew the kind of care he would receive. But no matter how good a hospital is, if the person isn't ready or prepared for it, the adjustment to such a change can be insurmountable.

I knew in my heart that he didn't have much time left now. I had seen this often enough to be able to make a prediction. Now his time on earth would be measured in weeks, not months. I couldn't help him. It was very difficult for me to accept this because I knew Ralph was happy where he had been for a year. He didn't want to cause any "trouble" for anyone. This abrupt decision to move him to a hospital so close to an accident, only confirmed to him that he was trouble for his family. Inside, I was angry as hell. I could, of course, never show my feelings or make any remarks that could be construed as judgmental. I had to hold my tongue and keep my emotions out of it. After the visit with Ralph and his daughter, I got as far as the curb, and when out of view, the social worker and I had a good cry. Ralph died two weeks later in the hospital. I want to believe he died peacefully, but I'll never know.

Your loved one doesn't want to be a burden. It is cruel at any time to let them think they are one. Please don't take a parent into your home and let him or her think this is where he or she can stay, and then pull the rug out at the last minute. My God, the suffering this causes is indescribable. Yet, this happens hundreds of times a day. Please be sensitive to your loved one's feelings.

My job is to prevent suffering, whether it be physical in origin or psychological. After the experiences I've had with the Ralphs of the world, I now tell families exactly what it is like to care for someone who is dying in the home. If they think they can't handle it, then I give them options. We make a plan with the patient. This way, everyone is prepared the way they should be. Here's what I tell them.

There are no horrendous death scenes to fear. If you can take a little throwing up occasionally, clean a soiled backside, give a bed bath, feed a meal, give an injection, turn the dial on the oxygen tank, help someone from their bed to the commode — that's almost all that is required. Caring for the dying is just that ...caring. It has more to do with giving of yourself than in the actual things you do. Caring for the loved one should be thought of as a privilege, not a chore. If you view it only as an obligation, then you should consider other alternatives. Caring out of obligation will not give you or your loved one what the experience is intended to give. It will only result in stress and resentment. If you're doing it out of love, it will bring you both happiness and peace.

Sure you're scared. You have to learn to give care. I still remember the first time I had to give an injection. That was many years ago! It's one of my favorite things to do now because it doesn't hurt and it makes my patients feel better. There is nothing more satisfying or more beautiful than coming into a situation where there is pain, a leaky colostomy, etc. and making things right. By the time I leave, all is well with the patient, the family, and my soul. I thank God every day I do a good job. You will thank Him too once you feel the love that comes back to you tenfold...when you care for someone you love.

So what options do you have when there is a six-month prognosis? It depends on the condition of the patient, insurance, and your financial resources. I'll describe two short situations, then an option or two.

Situation: Elderly Parent Lives Alone

Suppose your mother lives in an apartment some distance from you. She was given a prognosis of six months to live. These are your options:

- **You may want to ask her to come live with you.** If she decides to live with you, you could get home health care for her, provided she meets the criteria. Essentially, she must be homebound — which means she must be ill enough so that her condition prevents her from leaving her home, with the exception of going to see her doctor. She must have a "skilled need." A skilled need is one that requires the skill of a professional: a nurse, a physical therapist, an occupational therapist, or a speech therapist. Her physician must be the one to order home health care. If your mother has Medicare and is not in an HMO, home care services would continue as long as there is a medical need. If she is enrolled in an HMO, then home care may be discontinued because the HMO case manager may determine that a skilled need no longer exists, even though your mother's nurse may disagree.

- **You could have hospice care in your home.** Hospice is a special kind of home health care. Once you decide to have hospice care and they accept your case, then your mother's traditional insurance, if it is Medicare, converts to the hospice benefit of Medicare insurance. If she is in an HMO, the hospice benefit may be as many as 210 days per year with a co-pay, or as little as 125 days per year. The HMO contracts with a specific hospice agency. With traditional Medicare insurance or private insurance, you probably have a choice of several hospice agencies that are in your community. Hospice is special because there is a concerted team approach in the care of the patient and there is care for the family members. (In addition to offering counseling, hospice utilizes specially trained volunteers from the community to help in giving family members respite a few hours a week.) The hospice physician either becomes the patient's primary source of medical supervision or has a coordinating relationship with the patient's physician. Patients have expert care from medical professionals who specialize in end-of-life care. But hospice is more about learning how to live. I strongly recommend this approach for both patient and family.

- **You may choose to care for your mother without any outside help.** This is certainly your option as well as hers. The American Cancer Society and Cancer Care, as well as a host of other organizations, have a plethora of information for you. Caring for a patient or any other loved one on your own is difficult, but has some advantages. There would be a continuity of care, privacy, and the opportunity to bond more closely without external influences.

Situation: Elderly Parent Lives Alone and You Can't Help in the Care

Suppose your mother or father lived alone and because of your work situation and family obligations, you were unable to provide care.

- **You can obtain home health care for your parent in his or her own home.** However, there are certain criteria that have to be met that are different from the first situation described, in which he or she were in your home, and you were taking responsibility for him or her. The difference is this: patients living alone must demonstrate competency to be able to self-direct their care and they must be able to summon help in case of an emergency. They must be safe in their own home. For instance, if a person is prone to falls and has injured himself or herself in the past, a home health agency may refuse to accept the case because the patient would be viewed as unsafe.
In addition, patients must be able to take their own medication. If the patient is unable to prepare medication for himself or herself, then someone in the family or a close friend must be available to assist the patient.
Remember — home care is short term and intermittent care. It should not be regarded as a permanent solution to a long-term problem or situation.

If the patient is terminally ill, alone, and mostly bedbound, then it would be unsafe for this person to remain in his or her home, even with hospice care. How would he or she get a meal? What if there were a fall while attempting to get to the bathroom? How would he or she get washed? There would be a multitude of problems, and yet there are people like this living on their own. They will do anything to hang on to living in their own environment, even if it means crawling on the floor to get what they need. They are rigid in their determination to stay where they are. If you suggest a care facility or acute care hospice facility, they will flat out refuse. However, once they are gently introduced to the philosophy and care associated with these facilities, it becomes less threatening to the patient and sometimes, they will accept the change in environment.

Other Options

Nursing homes can contract with a community hospice program to bring the full range of hospice services to the terminally ill residing in the nursing home. The community hospice team would provide the care directly to the patient or in consultation with the nursing home staff.

All community hospice programs are designed to deliver services in the patient's home. There are very few facilities (hospitals/nursing homes) which are designated solely for hospice use. The ones that are dedicated to hospice use are facilities that are privately owned and operated. Some are operated by a religious order, like the Hawthorne Dominican Nuns who operate St. Rose's Home in New York City. Another hospital, Calvary Hospital in the Bronx, New York, is a 200 bed specialty hospital exclusively dedicated to the care of adult patients in the advanced stages of cancer.

Some community hospices have a collaborating agreement with a hospital that has an allocated unit for the use of homebound cancer patients. The hospice patient may need care in the hospital when death is imminent in one or two weeks, or for stabilization and symptom management. This allocated unit may also be used for providing the patient with care if the family needs a respite of up to five days.

People generally do better at home than in the hospital. Most people lose weight when they are in the hospital because it is stressful and they often don't like the food. It's not that hospital food isn't good, it just isn't what you get at home. Also, a hospital seems "threatening." It used to be the only place to go to die. Today most people still die in hospitals, because of several avoidable reasons

- **The family panics** when things turn for the worse. Of course, sometimes it is better to go to the hospital to stabilize the situation. I have sent people to the hospital because I knew they weren't ready to die and we needed short-term medical care from a physician who could only stabilize our patient in the hospital.

- **The family can't cope** with the end-stage care. Care in the end stage of the disease may need to be continuous. This is when sharing responsibilities and hiring outside help is needed to help cope.

- Physicians tend to keep the patient there for **opportunities to prolong life**, and to satisfy the family's need for respite. That need can become indefinite.

People do better at home because they have control over their environment. In contrast, there is no control in a hospital. There, you must wake up when they tell you to. Strangers come and go at their will, to poke, prod, invade, and command. If you have pain, you have to wait — sometimes in agony — until someone is convinced that, in fact, you are in pain. I can't tell you how many studies report the high incidence of pain in patients who are hospitalized. This says one thing to me. It means that pain is being largely ignored. There shouldn't be such a high incidence of ignored pain. Pain can be controlled 90 percent of the time.

People do better at home because they are surrounded by their "things" that represent safety and security, like their bed, or the reassuring pictures of parents and children with smiles held in time, as if to communicate the message that they are always with you, that you'll be all right. This is what dignity means.

Home health care can be a way to preserve your dignity and give you the care and support you need. You are loved by people around you. The love is just brought out better when it can happen in the right setting.

How Home Health Care Can Help All Cancer Patients

I could go into a discussion about the history of home health care and how many millions of visits are made each year, but I'm not going to do that. You need to know three things right now.

- What services can be provided to you.

- How long the services will be provided.

- Who will pay for the services.

First, let me just emphasize that home care can certainly take some of the burden away from the caregiver at a time when you need the most help. It can help by providing you with trained professionals who know how to maximize your loved one's potential for health and comfort. A home health aide (a paraprofessional) can take on the duties of providing personal care to your loved one, as well as the household chores of laundry, light housekeeping, cooking a meal, or shopping. This gives you, the primary caregiver, more time to rest and have more quality time with your loved one. You may also want to use this time for yourself to continue the activities you enjoyed previously, before this illness struck your family member.

You need some diversion from the continued stress of dealing with a dying loved one. You may want to use the time available to sleep. This helps to restore your energy, decrease stress, and increase your ability to cope.

Services Provided by a Home Health Care Agency

Under a Certified Home Health Care Agency (certified by the state), a multitude of services may be provided. All insurances use the Medicare guidelines for eligibility for services, as well as the Medicare criteria indicating the need for each service.

The services available include nursing visits, home health aide services, physical, speech, and occupational therapy, social worker visits, and provision of medical supplies and durable equipment.

My further discussion of these services will be in relation to the needs of the cancer patient or terminally ill patient only. Home care services can be provided for others with non-life threatening ailments, as well, but I wish to confine the discussion as it pertains to you.

Who Is Eligible for Home Care?

Anyone at any age is eligible for home care as long as you have insurance and:

- Patient is homebound — a patient is considered homebound if he or she has a condition that restricts his or her ability to leave the home except with the assistance of another.

- There may be an absence from the home as long as it is infrequent and of short duration — less than four times a month for only 2-3 hours each time.

- Patient must be under the care of a physician and have a signed order by the physician for home care services.

- Patient must require skilled nursing on an intermittent basis, or physical, speech, or occupational therapy. An intermittent basis means less often than daily and at least once within a 60-day period.

- Service must be reasonable and necessary. This means that the services provided are consistent with the severity of the illness. The treatment must be within acceptable standards of professional practice.

Skilled Versus Non-skilled Needs

The services described directly below are classified as skilled needs and are provided by medical professionals.
A skilled need is that which requires observation and assessment of the patient's condition. Descriptions of non-skilled needs are found further below.

Skilled Need:

- **Teaching and Training** — much of the patient's condition requires teaching and training. For example, if you have lung cancer, there could be a complication of fluid accumulation in the lung spaces or pleural lining. This is called pleural effusion. The nurse would have to observe your condition, teach you deep breathing exercises, show you how to take your own pulse rate, train you in energy conservation techniques, and instruct you on diet and emergency protocols. Another example of teaching and training would be teaching someone about ostomy care and training the person to perform the task on his or her own.

- **Administration of Medications** — for example, giving an intramuscular injection or intravenous drip infusion. The administration of oral medications or eye drops is not considered a skilled need.

- **Tube Feedings** — sometimes when a patient can't eat by mouth, the doctor may want to give feedings via a tube that goes into the stomach (called a percutaneous gastrostomy or jejunostomy tube).

- **Catheter Insertions** — in most cases, urinary catheter insertions require sterile technique and is a skill that the nurse performs. Family members are not expected to insert any foley or catheter.

- **Wound Care** — many times when a patient is bed bound, the skin breaks down and opens, creating a wound, or there may be a cancerous lesion that causes a wound. Care of wounds from burns, ulcers, pressure sores, or open surgical sites require the skill of the nurse to perform. A nurse may be required daily or up to twice daily to perform wound care. A patient or family member cannot be forced to learn wound care. If this is something you feel you cannot do - then the insurance company must pay for the service. If they do not, then you can appeal it. The criteria for giving a family member a task is that they must be willing and able to perform it.

- **Physical Therapy** — is a skilled need when the patient's condition will improve through therapy or when the services are needed to maintain the patient's condition. Maintenance programs are covered if a skilled therapist is needed to manage and periodically reevaluate the patient for safety and functional ability. Traditionally, the therapist evaluates the patient's present condition, formulates an exercise program, and teaches the patient/family how to maintain functional ability through therapeutic exercises.

    Normally, after a few weeks, the family members are able to supervise the patient in a home exercise program, which may consist of the proper way to get in or out of bed, increasing bed mobility tasks like turning and positioning, transfers from a bed to a chair, walking safely with a walker, and generally increasing the patient's strength and endurance.

    Many previously bedbound patients have progressed markedly in strength and independence due to the s kills of a good physical therapist, combined with the patient's own determination to live a better quality of life. Speech and occupational therapists work in the same manner.

Non-Skilled Need: The home health aide is the person who provides the patient with non-skilled services. He or she is a paraprofessional who has some training in personal care needs, including the safety and comfort of the patient. For home health aide services to be covered by insurance, these services must:

- Be reasonable and necessary to the treatment of the illness.

- Be part-time or intermittent.

- Provide hands-on personal care of the patient.

Personal care refers to bathing, grooming, dressing and hair care, feeding, assistance with elimination, assistance with walking, turning, positioning, and transfers. More specifically, the home health aide may:

- Measure input/output — take a temperature, pulse, or respiration reading, empty a catheter bag, cleanse the insertion site as directed by the nurse, assist by handing items to the patient used for wound care.

- Dispose of supplies and soiled dressings.

- Assist patient in colostomy care by handing items to patient, emptying colostomy bag.

- Assist patient in care of the skin with prescribed or over-the-counter medications, and/or non-medicated creams, powders, lotions, sprays.

- Assist with range of motion exercises.

- Assist with oxygen safety per a registered nurse's instructions.

The home health aide functions under the supervision of the nurse and has to follow a detailed care plan. The physical therapist may also supervise the home health aide.

There have been recent changes in the criteria used by insurance companies to determine home health aide placement and allowable hours. Not long ago, it was permissible to place an aide four hours a day for someone who is ambulatory but frail and who needs assistance with bathing and light housekeeping. Today, that same patient would perhaps only qualify for a two-hour aide for only three days a week instead of five. The primary use of the aide must be for personal care. If a patient can bathe and dress unassisted, then the aide is not needed and the insurance company will not approve the aide.

There are problems associated with this decrease in hours allowed. The vendors (home health care agencies) which supply the aide, often refuse to take a case because it is not cost-effective for them, when taking into account the travel time for the aide to get from one location to the next. (Most aides do not have cars and would have to use public transportation.) Vendors would rather have an aide placed four hours a day and might refuse to take a two-hour case by saying, "We don't have an aide for that area now." The patient often has to go without an aide for as long as 2-3 weeks until the case can be placed with another vendor.

Be prepared. When the hospital discharge planner discusses home care with you, he or she may promise you the moon, saying that you'll get an aide on the day after you are discharged. The fact is, you probably won't unless you are bedbound and need a lot of home health aide hours. Home health aides are mostly placed by vendors. Availability cannot be guaranteed.

The medical social worker is covered by insurance, provided these services are necessary to resolve social, emotional, or financial problems within the family that are an impediment to the effective care of the patient. For example, a patient with an altered body image or a terminal illness may need a social worker to provide counseling in coping techniques and stress reduction. The social worker can make referrals to community organizations that offer help with either financial, emotional, or manpower needs to assist the patient or family. If you cannot afford home care and you don't have sufficient insurance coverage, the social worker can help you apply for financial benefits through various entitlement programs.

Some HMOs have their own social workers on staff, so they may not approve the social worker visits from the Certified Home Health Agency (CHHA). The CHHA would have this information at the time of the referral. Nevertheless, a social worker will be provided if needed, whether from the CHHA or HMO.

What Does Part-time or Intermittent Mean?

Remember when I said that most insurances use Medicare criteria for eligibility for services? Well, Medicare covers either part-time or intermittent services.

- **Part-time means:** any number of days per week, up to and including 28 hours per week of skilled nursing and home health aide services combined, for less than 8 hours a day.

or

- up to 35 hours per week of skilled nursing and home health aide services combined, provided on a special case by case basis. The terminally ill patient who is bedbound qualifies.

This means that if you are bedbound and have a terminal illness, the nurse in charge of your care could put in any combination of nursing/home health aide visits he or she felt you needed (with the approval of your doctor). Suppose you needed more personal care than monitoring by a nurse. The nurse may place a home health aide for 4 hours a day, 7 days a week (28 hours), plus 2 one-hour visits by the nurse per week (30 hours total). There would still be 5 hours left which could be used to provide extra home health aide hours if the patient needed it.

- **Intermittent means:** up to 28 hours per week of skilled nursing and home health aide services combined, provided on a less than daily basis.

or

- up to and including 8 hours a day of skilled nursing and home health aide services, which are provided and needed 7 days a week for a temporary period of time up to 21 days.

While HMOs and other insurance carriers use the Medicare criteria for eligibility, they do not use the same hourly entitlement schedule. In other words, the patient must still be homebound and have a skilled need, but services are allotted according to their judgement, and this may differ from the judgement of the Certified Home Health Agency that is serving you. Since the HMO or other insurance company is paying your bill, it usually has the last word. If you want to contest its decision, you can do so by going through the process of appealing denials as outlined in Chapter Two.

Some HMOs have a co-pay, which the patient has to pay under their health services provisions. The co-pay ranges from $10.00 per visit to $20.00. In addition, most HMOs limit the number of home visits allowed in a year to 200, while others allow only 20 visits per year.

What would the services cost you if you didn't have insurance?

Nursing	Social Worker	Physical Therapist	Home Health Aid
$ 155.00	$210.00	$ 145.00	$100.00
Per Visit	Per Visit	Per Visit	Per Visit

Some agencies will provide services on a sliding scale basis. If you earned in the median yearly salary range of $36,000, nursing might cost you $62.00 per visit, social worker $84.00, therapist $58.00, and HHA $40.00. These figures are at 40 percent of the regular cost. Each agency has its own criteria for sliding scale.

Health care is very expensive any way you look at it. But it is far more cost-effective to have care provided for you in the comfort of your own home than it is in the hospital.

What You Should Know About Getting Good Care

There is a good side to everything in life as well as a bad side. You should be aware that most people are very satisfied with the care received from a home health agency. However, there are things you need to know to ensure that you are protected.

The Home Health Aide — He or she is either going to be an angel or someone you never want to see again. Sometimes it takes a bit of patience to find the right match for you. It could be a conflict of personality or a conflict of work ethics. Don't waste time. Don't keep someone if that person is aggravating you.

My Criteria for a Good Home Health Aide

- The person should be well-groomed and neatly dressed.

- The person should speak politely to you and ask if you need anything.

- The person should know what to do and get to it. Home health aides have to follow a written care plan from the nurse. It should be posted where he or she can refer to it. You should read it as well and complain to your nurse if he or she doesn't follow it.

- The person should work, not watch TV. A home health aide can and should be removed from your home if he or she watches TV. There is enough for them to do.

- The person should never be rude, offer opinions, or be disrespectful.

- The person should always have an identification badge on him or her.

- The person should be kind and gentle with the patient. Listen and watch how the aide behaves around your loved one. If it isn't with love, you don't want that aide.

- The person should be on time and stay the full contracted amount of hours. Don't accept stories of needing to leave early. Call the agency immediately and let the supervisor know. This is a common occurrence. The aide may say she has to go to the doctor or some other appointment. She stays an hour, has you sign the work sheet, takes three hours off, and gets paid for four!

What You Need to Do Before the Aide Comes

- Always protect your valuables. Put your jewelry in a safe place (not in the bedroom).

- Put your important papers away: checkbook, money, credit cards, etc. While it is noble to want to trust people, in this day and age, you can't. There are incidents of theft, so you need to protect yourself.

- Ask your loved one how he or she likes the aide. If he or she doesn't like the aide but you do, don't keep the aide. Your loved one may not want to tell you something that may have occurred. And life is too short to be unhappy with anything at this stage.

- Ask the agency which supplies the home health aide if they do criminal checks on their employees.

- Always write down the name of the aide and the agency he or she is from. Sometimes you may get a different aide on a certain day. You want to know who came and when.

I have had many cases where there were good aides. They can be a tremendous help to you. Often, there is a special bond that develops between the aide and the patient. Your loved one needs all the love and comfort he or she can get. Treasure that bond as a gift from heaven — there are real angels out there who work for little money and give a great deal of themselves in return. A good aide walks in as a stranger and leaves as part of the family.

How Long Will Service Be Provided?

It depends on the skilled need you have. If you have a wound that needs daily dressing changes and no one in the family can learn this, then the care will be provided until the wound heals. If you have cancer with a six month prognosis, you may not have a skilled need requiring a nurse to see you. However, if you have pain, or need monitoring for a condition that is worsening, then you have a skilled need. You could have home care intermittently, where services would continue until you get to a functional level. Then you would be "discharged" (service would cease). If you needed home care again at some later time, the process would then resume.

Who Will Pay for Home Care?

If you have insurance, your insurance carrier will pay for home care (possibly with a co-payment.) If you have straight Medicare, then Medicare pays without any co-payment. If you do not have insurance, then some home health agencies either have a sliding scale or a budget for charity. In order to get free service, a social worker would have to come to the home and do a budget work sheet, which has information about your income and expenses. If you don't have insurance and need the service, then this is a viable option for you. There are also hospices which care for the terminally ill at no charge. St. Rose's Home runs seven such hospices in New York City and upper New York State.

Planning Ahead

When someone you love is dying, time is of the essence in many ways. If life was hectic before this tragedy, it will be doubly so during. Cut things down to a minimum. Only do what is necessary. Make your lives as simple as possible.

There are things you need to do in the beginning. I am going to assume that you have a prognosis of six months or less. (Many people who have received this prognosis have long surpassed it, by as much as two years or more.) The truth is, no one ever really knows for sure. You need to take care of the following matters:

- If you are the patient, see your attorney together with your family. Make sure your legal affairs are in order.

- The person who is ill should have an advance medical directive and health-care proxy filled out (explained further below).

- Family members need to discuss with their loved one his or her consent to or request for the issuance of an order not to be resuscitated if this is what he or she wants. This is called a DNR order (explained further below.)

- Keep all your important papers (i.e. will) in a safe place but never in a safe deposit box, because the bank seals them once notice of death is received.

Advance medical directives are either a living will or a durable power of attorney. Either allow you to give directions regarding your medical care. An advance directive is important because:

- It protects your right to accept or refuse medical treat ment at a time when you may not be mentally or physi- cally able to communicate your wishes.

- It relieves the family of the responsibility of making difficult decisions on your behalf.

- It gives the physician guidelines in providing your care.

A health-care proxy gives a relative or friend the legal authority to make health care decisions for you when you are unable to do so for yourself. The health-care proxy is a legal document and enforceable in all states. Your local hospital and community home health agency has sample documents. Before executing a health-care proxy, make sure the person you are giving this power to is really willing to assume this responsibility.

The order not to resuscitate (DNR) means that the patient does not want health care providers to attempt cardiopulmonary resuscitation in the event of cardiac arrest or respiratory arrest. Cardiopulmonary resuscitation involves using drugs, electric shock, or pushing on the chest in an attempt to restart the heart and breathing. The DNR order has to be signed by the patient's physician at the request of the patient. A copy is kept in the home. It is important that the document be kept in an accessible area and its whereabouts known to everyone in the home. You can include the request for a DNR order in the advance directives.

How to Obtain the Services You Need

There are several ways in which you would or could be referred for home care. The first occurs when you are hospitalized. Your name, diagnosis, and room number is placed on a list. A discharge planner, who is either a social worker or a nurse, reviews your chart for criteria for home care. The nurse or social worker may be an employee of the hospital you are in or may be a staff member of the community home health agency that has a contract with the hospital. The discharge planner monitors your progress by reviewing your hospital records. He or she would then conference with your doctor and obtain an order for home care if deemed necessary. At some point, the discharge planner would visit you in your room and ask you if you are agreeable to having home health care services. If the patient is terminally ill and has not been visited by a discharge planner, ask to see one. If you are agreeable, then an initial nursing visit would be made within 24 hours of your hospital discharge.

The other method for referral would take place if you were already home and your doctor felt you would benefit from home care. Your doctor would need to call your community home health care agency and telephone the order to the intake department of the agency. The agency would then verify your insurance and obtain prior approval for an evaluation visit to assess the skilled needs. If your doctor does not bring up the issue of home care, raise the issue with him or her. Do not be afraid to ask or assume he or she thought about it.

Once on home care, there are strict mandates that the agency has to follow according to state regulations. Your chart is a legal instrument. You have a right to see your records and have them released to you once you are discharged from home care. This usually incurs a cost of about 75 cents a page. As a general rule, you should always ask for copies of your medical records. They are of great benefit when a new doctor or specialist sees you for the first time.

Whether you have home care through a Certified Home Health Agency, Licensed Home Health Agency, or through a hospice, care will be limited in terms of hours, services, and duration. Families generally have to supplement with their own time and financial resources if they want or need more care for their loved one.

The purpose of home care is to maximize a patient's level of independence and ability to function in their own environment. Due to a rise in the incidence of chronic and acute illness and constraints in insurance, people are being discharged from hospitals early and forced back into their homes while still in need of skilled nursing and therapy services. In response to this crisis, home care now provides high-tech services to an increasingly critically ill population. Complex hospital procedures like Total Parenteral Nutrition (intravenous nutrition), peripheral lines (intravenous lines), and mechanical ventilation (breathing machines), are now being performed in the home. This puts a tremendous demand on the families to learn skills that were traditionally reserved for nurses. Despite these drawbacks home care is still better than being in a hospital environment. At least at home, you have control over your environment. And there is no compromise in medical care if the patient is at home.

Home is where you want to be. If for any reason you cannot remain at home, then think about a hospice facility like Calvary or St. Rose's Home or something similiar in your state. The kind of care delivered to you in these special facilities is the next best thing to being home. These specialists in caring for the terminally ill are angels of mercy who truly understand your needs and concerns. You will be loved and respected and your hopes for maintaining your dignity will be fulfilled.

*   *   *   *   *

Speaking of dignity, the one sure thing that will erode away at dignity like acid, is pain. The next chapter is probably the most significant for you to read. Take it seriously. It could change your life and how you feel about yourself. This is where you and the family will learn to really take control. It's time to mount up like soldiers. This battle is real, with pitfalls, opponents, and sneak attacks. Pain is your enemy. If you don't learn how to fight it, it can kill your collective spirits, for the patient is writhing (needlessly) in pain, this can have a severe negative impact on the attitudes, outlooks, and lives of all the family members. We are not going to let that happen. All of you will now learn to take the path away from pain!

Chapter Six
A Path Away from Pain

Unhappy am I, because this has happened to me. Not so, but happy am I, though this has happened to me, because I continue free from pain, neither crushed by the present nor fearing the future. For such a thing as this might have happened to every man; but every man would not have continued free from pain on such an occasion.

Marcus Aurelius Antoninus

Almost all of us will experience severe pain at some point in our life. Our natural hope is that some compassionate physician will see our priority for relief as his or her priority to provide it. But unlike other medical problems, pain still remains largely untreated, and at best, treated ineffectively. The root cause of this problem stems from the fact that pain is a symptom, not a disease, and most medical professionals view symptoms as being subordinate to the treatment of disease.

If your physician is like most, he or she views pain as "to be expected given your medical condition." Truth is, these physicians are diverting the blame of pain to the disease and not to their own failure to provide adequate pain relief. It is also true that many physicians just don't know how to provide that relief. I know this because too many patients are given very weak drugs, which are not the standard medications for treating cancer pain.

In this chapter, the patient and the family will be given all the information needed to effectively co-manage pain. You will learn that most of your feelings about pain and pain medications are based on myths perpetuated by fear, anxiety, and hearsay. If you want yourself or a loved one to be pain-free, then you owe it to yourself to be brave and believe the truth about pain management. Push away any biases and preconceived notions because if you want to remain pain-free, that is what is required of you.

How important is it to be pain-free? For most people, it is priority number one. They would do anything to be free of pain. So would you.

I'm now going to tell you that you don't have to be in pain.

You don't have to cry and pray that someone will do something about it. We are going to do something about it right now. My dear friends, suffering isn't necessary. It isn't necessary for redemption, or punishment, or offerings. Neither is it necessary for you to be "snowed under" with drugs in order to be pain-free. You can get back to living again. You can be happy, eat, sleep, talk, smile, and laugh again. It is within your reach and there are dedicated health professionals out there who want to help you. The problem may be in finding them. Let me help in my way, by telling you what I know, and imploring you to seek the physicians who can free you from your pain: the oncologists, anesthesiologists, and pain specialists.

I do not believe in suicide or euthanasia, so we're not going to discuss that as an option. I truly believe that people who are forced to think along those lines are brought to their desperate thoughts by exhaustion from pain and an inability to cope with a quality of life that is unacceptable to them.

Quality of life is a relative term. What is quality to one person is unacceptable for another. But can that person whose quality of life was unacceptable transform his or her life into an acceptable quality? I think he or she can. For people to want to live, they have to be pain-free, feel useful and needed, and be happy and loved. There has to be a sense of purpose. People don't fight to die — they fight to live. That's your purpose. Fight to see sunsets, fight to teach your children something special. Teach them about life. Teach them about the courage you have had to live until now. It's pain that makes us want to die, and you can be living pain-free.

I would never give false hope. I would never promise what couldn't be delivered. I know that 90 percent of cancer pain can be controlled. That isn't my figure. That comes from the consensus of many experts in the field. There is one problem, however. You are probably not seeing a physician who can put you in that percentile.

Now I'm going to explain more fully why pain is a problem for so many people. Again, I have to say it has to do with your physician.

I have seen enough suffering to last a lifetime. For years, I have tried to understand the pervasive disregard and indifference by all too many medical professionals who shirk their responsibility for managing pain. The physician is the only one who has the power to write a prescription for a chemical compound that could bring peace and serenity to a body that is impaled with pain. Cavalier indifference has no place in the halls of honorable and ethical medicine.

Above all, do no harm — this is the physician's credo. Yet, allowing patients to live in a perpetual state of pain is harmful to both physician and patient. It is harmful to you, doctor, because it demeans you and your profession. It is harmful to your patients because it demeans their body, mind, and spirit. The effects of pain are profound enough to change a lover of life into a seeker of death. We cannot live without hope, even if the only hope we have is to be free of pain. Allowing pain is all about allowing harm.

Treatment of pain has become such a massive problem that it now requires specialists like oncologists and anesthesiologists to take on the responsibilities of the many physicians who are complacent about controlling pain. The time has long since passed for polite requests and respectful submissions. As I said, I've seen enough suffering to last a lifetime. That gives me the right to say, "What the hell are you doctors doing out there?"

Ninety percent of cancer pain is controllable, yet pointless, avoidable suffering continues. It will go on this way until the majority of medical professionals own up to their professional and humanitarian responsibilities. The information physicians need to know about pain control is clearly and concisely presented in the protocols of the American Pain Society and the Agency for Health Care Policy and Research. Everything physicians need to know about the medications and dosing schedules are in the pamphlets published by these organizations for the physicians' use. The knowledge a doctor needs to eliminate pain is as easy to obtain as making a phone call to either of these agencies.

Until you make that call it comes down to this: your patient will learn how to guide your writing hand into a respectful submission to their right to adequate pain management. It's a legal as well as an ethical issue. You can't use the excuse that medical school didn't provide pain management education, or that pain is normal given the disease process, or that patients are expected to have pain. Yes, patients will have pain at times, but it is your responsibility to ensure that it doesn't become a part of their everyday life. There are no excuses that physicians can give to the one million Americans who have cancer pain, when the medical literature emphatically states that 90 percent of patients can be pain-free. There are no excuses nurses can give to justify their failure to properly assess, report, and monitor pain and advocate on their patients' behalf.

The courts have held doctors and nurses responsible in the past for not providing adequate pain management. When more Americans know that the few who have taken their rights to court have won, we will see more professionals assuming a more active, responsible, respectful posture towards management of pain. It is regrettable that "Management of Pain 101" has to be taught in courts of law. You, the reader, will not have to take your rights to court. You just need to find a physician who is sensitive and responsive to pain management.

In Chapter One, I spoke about how attitudes of physicians, nurses, and families can prevent quality care from being delivered to patients. I spoke about how culture and bias play a role in our behaviors. It is these same cultural influences and biases which affect the way in which a patient's pain is managed and, most often, not managed. You, the patient and family, are going to need to understand this if you are going to take any responsibility for pain management.

As a general rule — never have blind faith or trust in a physician when it comes to pain management. Feel free to challenge his or her recommendations, especially if you're not getting relief. Have him or her give you the rationale for his or her course of action. You must have a knowledge of pain control so you can speak effectively and intelligently. You need to know whether the doctor's pain medication recommendation is reasonable. Later, I will teach you about the pain drugs, and when they should be prescribed, and you will know if and when you need to ask for a change in medication. These suggestions are based on accepted protocols from organizations that specialize in pain management. I will tell you more about these protocols later in Chapter Seven. I am convinced that this is the only way to ensure that you or your loved one can remain nearly pain-free.

Pain management should be effected as a team effort involving the patient, family, nurse, and physician. If there is a weak link, the team will fall apart. A team approach will work only if everyone is knowledgeable. Too often, the physician is the one who is resistant, not necessarily because he or she doesn't want to help. Often he or she doesn't know how to help. You may say, "how is that possible? He's a doctor!" I can tell you that in my experience and from reading mountains of literature, many doctors don't know. Let me give you one reason why this is so.

An internist or family practitioner usually has a practice of many different people who have a variety of different medical problems. Perhaps only a small portion of them have cancer. The internist or the general practitioner may or may not be aware of or have experience with the drugs or the specific protocols for pain management for cancer patients. Hence, the physician may underprescribe and/or may not feel comfortable changing a medication. Yet, that is what may be necessary to stay pain-free and lucid.

If you have a physician who is underprescribing, you will most likely remain in pain and feel that this is the way it has to be. Your immediate notion is that your physician knows best. Many physicians don't always know what is best. According to the book, *The Psychological Dimensions of Cancer*, the authors write that "Many physicians lack sufficient knowledge about pharmacology of analgesics and many providers, patients and family members hold a moral bias against taking medications, considering it an unacceptable sign of weakness" (Goldberg, Tull, 1983).[6]

The physician's lack of knowledge accompanied by the family's moral bias against using narcotics adds up to the patient not getting the necessary pain medication. In fact, the family's fear of narcotics is reinforced by the physician's reluctance to prescribe them. The "unacceptable sign of weakness" is really just a rationale to cover the fear of narcotics, as if strength of character should be the means to control pain. That is just not possible.

Let me, just for a minute, give you a mental picture of what it was like for me when I first became a member of a hospice team. Cases came to the team rapidly. Before long, there was a waiting list. Almost all of the team's patients were in pain. Do you remember seeing Gone with the Wind? There was a scene in the Atlanta railroad yard where at first the camera shows a small group of suffering soldiers on the ground, writhing in pain. Then, as the camera pulls back, you see hundreds and hundreds of wounded soldiers. All of them were suffering and there was no one to take care of them.

That is exactly what I saw in my mind's eye as I was confronted with one patient's agony after another. The scope of the problem was the same. In the beginning, I would accept a doctor's refusal to give a narcotic to his or her patient, even though it was clearly indicated. I would never accept that now. I have finally learned that doctors do not have all the answers. Aside from not knowing everything, their decisions are too often based upon factors that conflict with the patient's legitimate needs. For example, a doctor may not wish to prescribe controlled substances out of fear (misplaced) that he or she could lose his or her license (see below); or a doctor may not prescribe the optimum treatment because HMO guidelines mandate a "cheaper" procedure or drug modality. (Most HMOs do not cover the cost of pain management through a specialized pain center, as in a pain clinic that is separate from a hospital). Let's look at some facts:

- On the average, 75 percent of patients with advanced cancer have pain. 40-50 percent report moderate to severe pain and 25-30 percent report severe pain (Jacox, A., Carr, DB, Payne, R., et. al 1994).[9]

- Pain is always subjective. (It is what you say it is.)

- Physicians, nurses, patients, and family members fear addiction, and this is the major reason for undertreatment.

- Abundant study data demonstrates the contrary — addiction is rare when opiates are used for pain management.

- Ninety percent of cancer-related pain can be adequately controlled.

- All patients with moderate pain or greater should be treated with an opiate drug.

- "...DEA (Drug Enforcement Agency) has consistently emphasized and supported a physician's authority to pre-scribe, dispense or administer them (pharmaceutical controlled substances) when indicated for a legitimate medical purpose."*

- "The CSA (Controlled Substance Act) does not set forth standards of medical practice, nor does it limit the quan-tity of a controlled substance that may be prescribed. It is the responsibility of individual practitioners to treat patients according to their professional judgement in accordance with generally acceptable medical standards."*

- "A physician need not fear DEA action or sanction if he prescribes controlled substances for a legitimate medical purpose within the usual scope of professional practice."*

* Letter from U.S. Department of Justice, Drug Enforcement Administration to author dated February 4, 1999. (See Appendix 7)

Why You Have Pain

We know that 75 to as much as 90 percent of patients with advanced cancer have pain. What causes this pain? Cancer pain comes from tissue damage as a result of cancerous lesions invading normal tissue, organs, and/or bone. What's called *visceral* pain comes from internal organs in the body, primarily in the abdominal cavity. *Somatic* pain, on the other hand, comes from inflammation or damage to subcutaneous, or deep tissue. Common causes of somatic pain include damage or inflamation caused by bone metastasis, liver metastasis, and biliary, bowel, or ureteral obstructions. Visceral pain can be dull, aching, cramping, or burning. Somatic pain is dull, aching, throbbing. There is also *neurogenic* pain (neuropathic) which is tingling, burning, or sharp and is associated with nerve compression or damage to nerves.

Drug therapy is aimed at interrupting the pain signals to the brain. Most drug interventions control all three types of pain at the same time. Sometimes a drug modality may not be effective in controlling *neuropathic* pain, which may require a more selective form of management, like a nerve block. I'll discuss treatments a little later in Chapter Seven.

According to the International Association for the Study of Pain, "Pain is the unpleasant sensory and emotional experience associated with actual or potential tissue damage." Pain is perceived via a complex system of signals and messages delivered to the brain.

These signals travel via free nerve endings in the skin, internal tissues, arterial walls, and joint surfaces, as well as in the brain. These free nerve endings, or pain receptors, can be stimulated by mechanical, thermal, or chemical means.

The mechanical stimulation of the pain receptors comes from tissue ischemia — a lack of blood flow causing a lack of oxygen as well, since oxygen is carried within the red blood cells. This ischemia can be caused by mechanical compression of tissues. For instance, when you sit for long periods of time, you can develop pain in the buttocks because of compression not only on the nerves, but on tissues. People who are bedbound and who do not reposition or turn themselves develop bedsores — mechanical stimulation of the pain receptors results.

Thermal stimulation of the pain receptors occurs with extreme temperature, either hot or cold. The pain associated with severe sunburn is an example of this.

Then there is the chemical stimulation of the pain receptors. We have chemical stimulators in our bodies that excite the pain receptors. These chemicals are bradykinin, serotonin, prostaglandins, acids, potassium ions, as well as some others. These chemicals are formed in tissues when there is damage to tissues, and these chemicals stimulate the pain nerve endings.

Pain is actually transmitted from the nerve endings to the brain through the control centers of the spinal cord. It travels from these control centers to the brain via two special pathways. When the brain receives the message, you then "feel" the pain.

The different drug modalities, especially the opiate drugs (narcotics), act to block pain by binding to opiate receptors in the body. This action inhibits further transmission of the pain signal. Opiates provide their effect in the spinal cord as well as at the body's opiate receptor sites. There are opiate receptor sites in the bowel, and in the pons and medulla of the brain. Opioid drugs are the drugs of choice for treating cancer pain.

Addiction Versus Tolerance

There is a natural resistance in our society to taking opiate medications because of the widespread stigma against narcotics in general. We associate narcotics with street use. The negative connotations of "drug heads," "dealers," and the like make it difficult to see the redeeming value of a drug that is so feared and exploited. This bias extends into the medical community, where the value of opioids are known, yet physicians are strongly resistant in prescribing them for their patients.

An important study reported in the *New England Journal of Medicine* in 1980 concluded that addiction is rare in patients treated with opioids/narcotics. Out of 11,882 patients given a narcotic drug treatment, only four became addicted (Porter & Jick, 1980).[14] There have been many subsequent studies which all conclude that addiction is rare when narcotics are given for pain. Studies have shown that in a total population of 24,000 patients, only 7 could be documented as becoming addicted as a result of receiving a narcotic for pain relief (Friedman, 1990).[5] Addiction is a psychological dependence on a drug characterized by an uncontrolled craving for the substance. The compulsive dependence on the drug is for the effects other than pain relief.

Addiction is sometimes confused with increasing drug tolerance. Tolerance means that a larger dose of opioid analgesic is required to maintain the original effect. The first sign of the development of tolerance may be a decrease in the duration of effective analgesia, according to the American Pain Society booklet *Principles of Analgesic Use in the Treatment of Acute Pain and Cancer Pain*, (pg. 25). Tolerance should not be confused with addiction. The body becomes accustomed to a certain dose and the analgesic effect decreases. Most often, a change in dose is needed to control the pain. This is a common occurance. Once there is stabilization of pain/analgesic effect, there is no further need to increase the dose.

It is important to remind you that there is no limit or ceiling on the amount of an opioid a patient may require. As long as doses are gradually increased, with a waiting period to monitor pain relief effects, a patient can receive as much as is required to relieve pain.

I have had patients on morphine who required 1,000 mg./day. Reports have indicated that patients have needed as much as 10,000 mg./day. The usual starting dose is 10-30 mg./every four hours or 15-30 mg. extended-release tablets every 8-12 hours. My patients who were on 1,000 mg./day were able to be titrated down when the pain decreased.

It doesn't matter what specific dose you are on. What matters is that your pain is being controlled. There should be no limit or ceiling to the amount of narcotic medication you are given as long as it is metered carefully and in increments, starting from the lowest dose and incrementing up as needed to control the pain. Of course, you should never stop taking your medication abruptly. This will cause withdrawal symptoms.

Common Concerns

* **Being Labeled**
  Many people will not approach the subject of their pain with either the doctor or their family. They don't want to be labeled a complainer and they don't want to be a burden. The result is unnecessary suffering in silence.

  Please, you must tell someone about your pain. You will not be labeled a complainer. Though not all doctors have a full understanding of how to treat cancer pain, they do understand that it is real. This is when you need to start becoming your own advocate. You can start by talking about your pain to your doctor, family, or nurse. Your pain is real and it can and should be controlled at the onset.

* **Worsening Pain**
  What happens if the pain gets worse? People fear that if they start on morphine, there won't be anything else to do if the pain worsens. This is not true. Usually, when pain increases, the dose of the opioid is adjusted to control the pain. Sometimes what helps one person may not be helpful to another. In this case, there may be a change in drug choice. It would still be an opioid, but a different one. Very often though, all that is needed is an increase in dose. The increase may be 25 percent more or it could be 50-100 percent more. The guidelines suggest 50-100 percent more for the non-elderly patient, depending

on the severity of the pain. It is possible to control the pain even if pain worsens.

- **Will the medication make me sleep all the time?**
  No. It shouldn't. Initially, when a first dose is given, you may be sleepy for the first day or two. Then your body adjusts to the medication. You should be able to have a normal day after the adjustment period of one or two days. Some medications affect people differently. Almost all patients remain alert and oriented.

- **Will I ever be able to go off the medication?**
  Yes, sometimes this can be accomplished when you receive radiation therapy or chemotherapy. Radiation therapy is often used to treat cancer pain and nearly 50 percent of patients have pain relief with this method.

- **What about the side effects from using opioid medication?**
  The most common side effects are constipation, nausea, and dizziness. You should be on a bowel regimen which includes stool softener or a mild bulk laxative (ask your doctor). Nausea can be controlled with the measures outlined in Chapter Three.

There is always some respiratory depression when taking an opioid medication. This means that respirations (breathing) slow down. Normal repirations are 12 to 18 breaths per minute in the normal resting adult. Clinically significant respiratory depression is rare, but may occur in elderly patients who are already compromised with a poor respiratory status. Careful monitoring is always the rule, especially when doses are changed or with the initiation of a new or different medication that has an effect on the respiratory system. The way to monitor respiratory function is to count the number of times the person's chest rises in one minute or the number of inhalations in one minute. If respirations are below normal, then careful and frequent monitoring is necessary. Check with your doctor on when he or she wants to be called when respirations are decreased.

Biased Attitudes

There is no question — if anything is going to prevent you from being pain-free, it is the biased attitudes of almost everyone who is in contact with you. Earlier, I mentioned how people bring their past experiences, culture, and attitudes into their practice of medicine and health care. You, yourself, as well as your family members have your own culture-specific beliefs that affect how you communicate with each other and others. This is demonstrated not only in what you say, but also in what you don't say; in what you do, as well as in what you don't do.

The same will be true for your health care providers. The doctor for instance may say, "I have to be careful what I give you because narcotics are regulated by the DEA, (Drug Enforcement Agency)." This is not a valid reason because in the words of one agent I spoke with at the DEA, "Narcotics are never an issue for us when it comes to prescribing them for cancer pain." The doctor is passing on his judgmental attitudes towards narcotics because of his beliefs and lack of appropriate knowledge. This fear is then passed on to you. Many times, a doctor will write an order for an opioid medication "p.r.n.", which means "as needed," when all the guidelines say the medication has to be given around the clock (whether it is every 4,8, or 12 hours) to avoid peaks and valleys of pain. If the medication is prescribed "as needed," the patient is forced to beg for the medication. This should never be. When an opioid medication is prescribed for you, **IT MUST BE AROUND THE CLOCK!**

Strong put it best in her article in *Nursing 92* where she stated, "Study after study clearly shows that we underestimate our cancer patients' pain and that most nurses rate a patients' pain by external signals rather than the correct way — by relying on what the patient tells them" (Strong, 1992, Pgs. 47-49).[19] In fact, nurses are not likely to come to a patient's rescue unless the patient shows highly visible signs of being in distress. They respond more to groans and screams. If the patient doesn't act like they're in pain, then the common assumption is that they're not in pain. But this is a very serious mistake in judgement.

We know that patients often use humor, sleep, or isolation to cope with pain, yet nurses fail to recognize these coping mechanisms and this results in the patient not getting the medication he or she needs. If the patient is sleeping, the nurse won't wake the patient up. If the patient is laughing, it is not likely that the patient will get his or her pain medication. It's a "You have to show me" kind of situation which is extremely demoralizing and humiliating for the patient.

Be firm. Tell the nurse, "Listen to what I am saying: I'm having a lot of pain." I'll tell you more about this later, but what you have to learn to do is rate your pain. It's called the pain scale rating system. On a scale of 0-10 (O means no pain, 10 is the worst possible pain), give your pain a number rating: "My pain is a level 8, on 0-10 scale. I need my medication now." If you don't get satisfaction, then ask to speak to the nursing supervisor or your doctor. Make a complaint.

The nurse's assessment of pain is influenced by her or his own ideas of what the behavior and emotional reaction of the patient should be. If a patient complains too much, then they are labeled "a problem patient." This is exactly what a patient is afraid of. You would never be referred to in such a manner by people who know and understand your suffering. And believe me, there are many thousands of professionals who do understand, and take your pain very seriously.

What about biased attitudes of your family members? Your family has fears that you would become addicted. I can understand this because of all the negative press narcotic use gets in the papers, movies etc. Your family has not been exposed to the medical uses of narcotics. It is easy to develop a blanket fear or believe a blanket statement when you have no proof to the contrary. But there is proof to the contrary.

Your family just doesn't know about it, nor has anyone taken the time to explain it to you.

A fear of narcotics is just one factor that can prevent you from getting the pain management you need. There are many such variables — I've counted eighteen of them! One day I began to systematically identify all the behaviors and attitudes of the people connected to the patient, as well as those of the patients themselves. What follows is my own theory and model for keeping patients pain-free. I call it **The Continuum of Pain, The Continuum of Pain Control.**

One morning in 1993, at 5 A.M., I was sitting at my kitchen table. My hair was askew and I was wearing mismatched pajamas, no doubt a reflection of my state of mind. I had spent months identifying the different influences that affect the patient's access to adequate pain control. I found myself staring at the sugar bowl and a glass that was next to it. After what seemed to be a long while, my left hand moved the bowl to the left, my right hand moved the glass to the right. Taking a pen and paper, I traced a circle around each object. As I sat and stared at the two separate circles, the floodgate opened. My writing had a hard time keeping up with the information that was racing through my mind. When I finished, I had the conceptual model for my theory: The Continuum of Pain, The Continuum of Pain Control. Side by side, each circle was like a mirror image of the other, yet distinctly different. The circles contained the object of interest, pain on the left, pain control on the right.

There are four groups involved in the pain circle and these same four are involved in pain control: the patient, physician, family, and nurse. On the continuum of pain, there are eighteen negative factors which contribute to pain. Eleven of these are general factors, which influence the continuum of pain but are not directly responsible for the continuation of it. Seven are absolute factors, which are directly responsible for the existence of pain. You only need one absolute factor out of the seven to keep pain going on in the continuum. Let's take a closer look.

Continuum of Pain
Non-Interdependent
Non-Facilitators

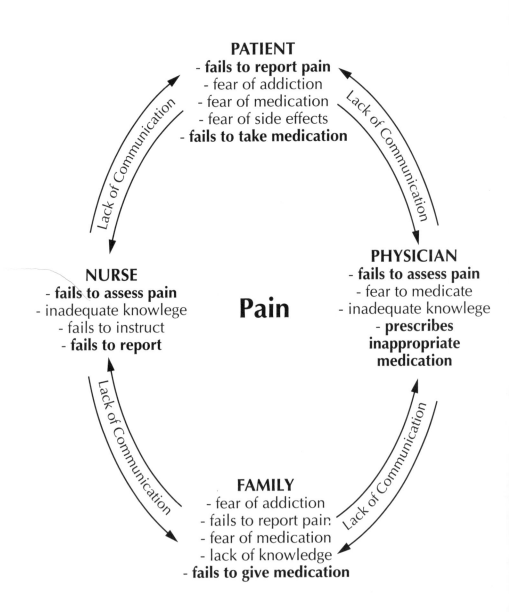

Please Note: Bold items signify absolute factors
© 1993 Nancy Hassett

Continuum of Pain Control
Interdependent Roles
Facilitators

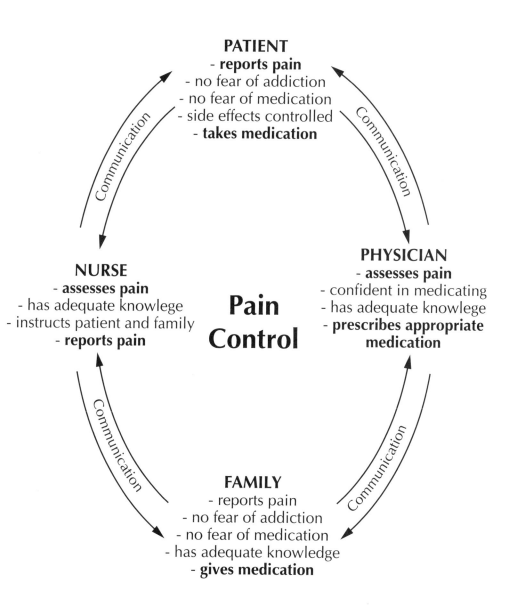

Please Note: Bold items signify absolute factors
© 1993 Nancy Hassett

The Continuum of Pain

The general negative factors that are associated with the **patient** include fear of addiction, fear of the medication, and fear of side effects — these all contribute to pain because they may influence how, when, and if the patient will take his or her medication. However, the two absolute factors — failure to report pain and failure to take medication — will absolutely keep that patient in a state of pain.

The general negative factors associated with the **nurse** include inadequate knowledge, and a failure to instruct the patient/family in medication use, dosage, schedule, and side effects. These all contribute to, but are not directly responsible for, the continued pain. However, if the nurse fails to assess the patient's pain or fails to report pain to the physician, these are absolute factors and will definitely be responsible for continued pain.

The general negative factors in the **family** are the fears of addiction, failure to report pain, fear of the medication, and lack of knowledge of the medication. These all contribute to pain. There is only one absolute factor associated with the family: failure to give the medication. The general negative factor of failing to report pain can become an absolute factor for the family if the patient (for whom reporting pain is an absolute factor), is unable or unwilling to do so. In this case, the patient's absolute factor of failing to report pain transfers to the family's responsibility and converts that general factor to an absolute factor. Since many patients are dependent on family members administering the medication, if they fail to do this, the patient will have pain.

The general factors associated with the **physician** are a failure to assess the patient's pain, fear of medication, and inadequate knowledge. There is one absolute factor — prescribing inappropriate medication. We don't need the physician to assess the pain — the nurse can do this. His or her fear of the medication in terms of side effects, addiction etc., may influence how he or she prescribes. But if he or she prescribes the inappropriate medication, the patient will definitely remain in pain.

The continuum of pain is an overall non-interdependent relationship among the people who are all non-facilitators in managing pain. The continuum exists and is perpetuated by a lack of communication in all directions. On this entire continuum, you only need **one** absolute factor to keep the pain going.

Continuum of Pain Control

The continuum of pain control is the exact opposite of all those factors, both general and absolute, that are found on the continuum of pain. However, there is a distinction — it is not an inverse relationship. The significant weight of the factors or their ability to influence is different in each continuum. This means that if one absolute factor moves over from the control continuum to the pain continuum, it **won't stop pain** from continuing. For instance, if the physician gives the appropriate medication (pain control) but the family fails to give it, the patient will have pain. It would take **all** the absolute factors from the control side to move over to the pain side to maintain the patient pain-free. However, you only need **one** absolute factor from the continuum of pain to stop pain control. It would stop pain control like a cog placed in the spokes of a wheel.

The continuum of pain control functions within the dynamic exchange of interdependent roles and everyone is a facilitator in maintaining the patient pain-free. There is communication in all directions between everyone. There is a definite team approach that is supportive and interactive. The patient is maintained pain-free in this continuum. It becomes a win, win, win situation. The patient wins because he or she is happy and can function at a higher level. The family wins because they feel a sense of accomplishment, relief, and equilibrium. The doctor wins because the patient and family are grateful and appreciative. Harmony, happiness, hope, and equilibrium abound in this continuum.

This is how I managed patients in pain. Nearly 90 percent were kept at pain levels of 0-3 on the 0-10 pain scale. This means that they experienced no pain to mild pain because I ensured that only the positive factors were in place within the continuum of pain control. The family and patient can do this by monitoring the negative factors on the continuum of pain and preventing them from moving over to the control side.

Another very important tool in keeping a person pain-free is the use of the pain scale rating system. This is absolutely necessary to keep the patient, your loved one, from having pain.

Pain Scaling

There have been different pain scales published by different organizations, two of which appear below. The most widely used system is the number scale (Numeric Pain Intensity Scale), 0-10. Zero is no pain, 5 is moderate pain, and 10 is the worst possible pain.

0-10 Numeric Pain Intensity Scale

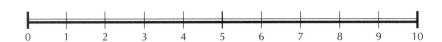

Simple Descriptive Pain Intensity Scale

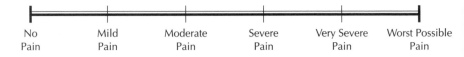

I find that patients do better with the numeric scale, because it doesn't require them to have to think. Pain scaling is the most effective tool in assessing a patient's pain level. It gives us a lot of information. For example, if a patient was at level 2 yesterday and today is at level 8, I know something is very wrong: Did she take this morning's dose? What level was she at at the time of taking her dose? This is six hours later. She's not due for two more hours. I give her the medication and call the doctor. We increase the dose but keep the same hourly spread. I always call the patient one to two hours later to get another pain scale rating and I chart it. I inquire as to how she's feeling and make another visit the next day. If she remains at a level 0-2, I am satisfied.

The family members are also taught to use the pain scale. We keep a flow sheet record in the home. Whenever pain is assessed, it must be done with a pain scale, and if it is at a level 5, it has to be reported to the family, nurse, or doctor as a number rating. This is the only way we can determine how severe the pain is. Otherwise it is just a word — pain. That doesn't give us enough information. The doctor adjusts the medication according to the number you rate your own pain. No one else can do this. Only you know what number to assign to your pain.

We also assess pain in terms of duration and intensity. How long does it last? What quality does it have? Is it burning, sharp, dull, throbbing? Does it move from one place to another or is it confined to one area? Is there anything you do that helps it? Be ready to answer these questions before you call.

The physician needs a good mental picture and pain scale rating to determine the appropriate medication. A few pages below, you will see an example of the flow sheet I use when I have a patient in pain. This is from an actual patient's report of pain. You can see how the pain fluctuated. We try to keep the pain level at 0-2. A moderate level, which is 5, requires the use of an opioid if the level remains at 5. The flow sheet shows large gaps of dates. This means the patient has remained stable until the next incidence of pain, which required necessary action. You can see that the medication needed to be changed on 10/12. His pain level came down quite a bit until 11/21, when he reported a marked increase in pain, which he had for most of the day. The medication was again adjusted. He remained at levels 2-3 until 12/28. He was then sent to the clinic where a different doctor took him off the morphine and put him back on Tylenol #3. His pain was again high at 7-8. He was admitted to the hospital briefly for pain management. His pain level came down to 3-2 until he ran out of medication. Then the pain shot up to level 10 — the worst pain. Once the prescription was filled and he resumed his medication, the level came back down to 2. He remained at that level for months.

The reasons for the fluctuation in pain are attributed to several factors. On 10/11 the nurse failed to assess the patient's pain. On 11/21 it was evident that the patient had developed a tolerance to the dose given 10/12 so the medication needed to be increased. On 12/28, the patient again developed increased pain. This increase may be due to the disease process or attributable to a tolerance effect. On 12/29 the patient's pain stayed high because the narcotic was discontinued by a physician who was unfamiliar with the patient. **Absolute Factor**: physician prescribes inappropriate medication.

The other increases of pain were due to lack of planning. The patient/family/nurse allowed the medication to run out before getting a new prescription. **Factor**: nurse's inadequate knowledge and failure to instruct the patient/family on the importance of monitoring medication for sufficient quantity to prevent a pain crisis. **Factor**: family — lack of knowledge. **Absolute Factor**: patient — fails to take medication because there is no medication. **Result**: Pain. You will not experience the dramatic fluctuations shown in the example if the Continuum of Pain Control is strictly adhered to. And, there is another lesson to be learned from this case. Since pain control is a delicate balancing matter, it is unwise to let any physician other than your primary provider of pain-control alter or change the medication you receive for pain.

PAIN SCALE FLOW SHEET (0-10 SCALE)

| Patient | Date of Initial Evaluation |

Tylenol #3   2 Tabs q 6 HRS PO

Current Analgesic Prescribed

| Doctor | Phone Number |

DATE	TIME	PAIN RATING	MEDICATION CHANGE	R*	P**	SIDE EFFECTS/COMMENTS
8/31	Noon	0	No Change			0
9/29	3PM	0	No Change			0
10/11	10AM	No Rating		18	90	Nurse feels Pt in pain - No scale done
10/12	10AM	7	MS Contin 30mg q12***	18	90	Pain right hip, shoulder doctor called
10/13	8:30	5				Not eating - not taking meds on time
10/14	11AM	3				Eating, taking meds - No N/V
11/21	2PM	9-10	MS Contin 30mg q8	20	84	Increased pain - MD called - new dose.
11/22	10AM	7		20	92	Pt sitting up alert, pain in AM only
11/23	11AM	3				Sleeping well, eating
12/28	10AM	7-8		24	80	Pt cries in pain per spouse sent Pt to clinic today
12/29	9AM	7-8	Tylenol #3 2 Tabs q4			MD did not renew Ms. Contin - Called Dr.
	12 Noon	10				Dr. Smith - request HOS Admission
1/6	10AM	3	MS Contin 60mg q8	18	76	Dr. Smith to manage
1/27	10AM	2	MS Contin			

* Respiration
** Pulse
*** MS Contin is morphine sulphate (extended release morphine)

Conclusion

Now you can see that pain management requires diligent tracking. Side effects should be noted in the right-hand column and respiration and pulse should be monitored as well, especially when a new dose of medication is introduced. I usually ask patients and/or family members to do a pain scale rating prior to taking the medication and one hour after. A pain scale rating should be done about three times a day by the family. If the pain rating is 5 or greater, call the doctor. Report the pain rating your loved one has given you. For example: "Doctor, John is having increased pain. On a 0-10 scale, he is reporting a level 5 pain, which he has had all day. Nothing seems to relieve it."

You can't and shouldn't rely on the nurse to do a pain scale rating. Many nurses are not familiar with using it and because pain requires frequent tracking, the best way is for you to do it. You'll know when the pain medication is effective by evidence of a low pain scale rating (0-3) on a 0-10 scale.

The effects of pain are far reaching and profound. Pain can cause depression, sleeplessness, agitation, despair, and hopelessness in both the patient and the family. The effects of pain can destroy any efforts toward maintaining dignity and lead a person to think that dignity can only be found through the cessation of life.

Quality of life is very much dependent on the quality of pain control. Hope, love of family, enjoyment of food, music, reading, laughter — all these can only exist in a pain-free environment. This is why pain management must be everyone's priority. It is the one precious gift we give that returns the many other gifts of seeing our loved one enjoying life with us.

Pain management is everyone's responsibility. Since 90 percent of cancer pain can be controlled, we should set our goal to be in that 90 percent group. The patient's responsibility lies in self-assessment, using the pain scale rating system, and in reporting the pain. The result of not reporting pain puts an undue burden of suffering not only on the patient, but on the family members who have to watch the patient suffer in silence. This in turn causes tremendous grief, despair, and anger for the family members because it leaves them feeling powerless. (This is when they must take on the patient's absolute factor of reporting the pain.) The secondary result is a division of patient/family values, trust, and cohesiveness — the continuum of pain control and the family unit itself both fall apart.

The family's responsibility in pain management is to encourage open communication. The family is better equipped to monitor for pain and side effects than the patient. The family is not as affected by the changes in physiological disruptions as the patient is. As a family member, though you are influenced by fear, stress, and possibly depression, your mental capacity and physical strength put you in a stronger position to manage your loved one's pain. This means pain scaling and charting on a flow sheet, reporting the pain to the physician, making sure there is enough medication, and planning ahead so it doesn't run out. It may also mean giving the medication if your loved one isn't able to self-medicate. You should give the medication on time and around the clock as your physician has prescribed it, never PRN as needed. The family is the pivotal key in good pain control.

The nurse's responsibility (he or she has many during a visit, but only the pain aspect will be addressed here) is to also assess for pain in a clinical manner, including pain scaling and physical assessment. He or she should also institute a pain scale flow sheet, and any pain that is not acceptable to the patient should be reported to the physician immediately. The nurse should instruct the patient/family in the use, dosages, and side effects of the medication(s) and ensure that there is an adequate supply. The nurse can be a valuable support and source of information. He or she very often shares in the intimate emotions and concerns of those entrusted to his or her care. It is common, however, for nurses to neglect the full extent of this responsibility for pain management. And because it must be done by someone, this is why the information is here for you...so you can take charge.

The physician's responsibility is to provide adequate pain management by prescribing and continuously evaluating the appropriate medication, and providing support and explanations for the basis of choosing one modality over the other. This responsibility includes review of the literature that supports the widely accepted protocols established by government and non-government agencies and societies. Comfort, compassion, knowledge, and appropriate action are the indicators for what is honorable and responsible. If your physician isn't comfortable doing the pain management, then seek an oncologist, anesthesiologist, or go to a pain clinic. But in the meantime, give your physician the resources that are meant for him or her to use (see Chapter Seven).

Pain management is possible, in the presence of a systematic approach. Pain should be a signal that initiates a very specific set of actions, not unlike when a code is called in the hospital. In a code situation, the team is rallied. Everyone knows their function. A quick assessment is made and the protocol begins. Pain should elicit the same team response:

Step 1 Assessment — Description of the pain: intensity, duration, contributing factors, pain scaling. Effects of the pain: sleep, appetite, physical activity, concentration, emotions.

Step 2 Examination of the factors — Does everyone know their part? (Continuum of Pain Control)

Step 3 Initiate the protocols -

1. Pain is reported based on the assessment.
2. Medication regime is established.
3. Evaluation of effectiveness.
4. Ongoing monitoring of the response.
5. Ongoing monitoring of possible side effects.

If pain is still present, return to Step 1.

Keep in mind:

- Addiction is rare. Studies have shown that in a tota population of 24,000 patients, only 7 could be documented as becoming addicted as a result of receiving a narcotic for pain relief (Friedman, 1990).[5]

- Pain management requires a team approach involving the patient, physician, family, and nurse.

- Rating the pain with the numeric pain scale is your most important tool in controlling pain.

- You must tell someone about your pain.

- 90 percent of cancer pain can be controlled. The other 10 percent can be helped in some cases with intraspinal administration of morphine. Consult your oncologist or anesthesiologist.

*　*　*　*　*

You are now well on your way to mastering pain control. As you can see, the medication prescribed is just a part of the process. With the proper medication, you will find that you will be able to enjoy life again. Take comfort in knowing that there are thousands of health care professionals committed to the well-being of all cancer patients and working to improve your quality of life. You are part of us all. And we are responsible for one another.

This is the first half of the Path Away from Pain. The second half will deal with the common medications that are prescribed for each level of pain. Every patient is unique. What has been effective for one patient may not be effective for another. Only a physician who knows the protocols can prescribe the medication you need. Chapter Seven will give you a general picture of the medications that are usually prescribed for cancer pain.

Chapter Seven
A Path Away from Pain - the Medications

It is not fit that I should give myself pain, for I have never intentionally given pain even to another.

Marcus Aurelius Antoninus

Think of your life in terms of what it could be, not what you think it has to be. Lying in a darkened room with the covers pulled over your head is not living with quality. You could be sitting at the kitchen table enjoying a home-cooked meal. You could be bantering with family members about who remembers what best. A whole lifetime could be relived in a matter of months. A new sense of self could emerge from the strength that troubled times bring. You have choices.

Believe it or not, the choice of taking pain medication is often not an easy one. Many people choose not to take the medication, take it only once in a while, or take something ineffectual from their medicine cabinet, knowing it will not help. Some people pride themselves on not ever taking anything medicinal. Some offer their suffering as a sacrifice in the hope of forgiveness for past sins. Some refuse medication in order to elicit attention from those who were previously inattentive. Others fear that taking the small pill will force them into an existence of nonbeing, non-knowing and/or non-caring. The reasons are as limitless as they are wrong.

What a joy it is to discover that something you thought was wrong could be so right. The only regret ends up being that of lost time. And time is something none of us can afford to lose.

I want you to live your life as you have lived it until now. I want you to appreciate the gifts of life that are meant for you to enjoy. You have suffered enough in your lifetime, through all the trials and tribulations that come to all of us. This latest choice of suffering need not be made. On the contrary, it is honorable to acknowledge and respect your body by protecting it from harm and suffering.

Pain medication will help you be yourself again. It will lift your spirits, ease your anxiety, and allow hope to replace hopelessness and despair. It is entirely your choice. The gift your loved ones bring you is being there for you. The gift you bring your loved ones is being there for them. Pain medication can help you do this.

The medications used for pain management are only a part of the process of controlling pain. Attitudes, receptiveness, coping abilities, and know-how are all factors which determine success. Every patient is different and this means that a specialized regimen must be created to suit the needs of any one particular person. What works for one may not work for another. To achieve sustained pain relief, an ongoing assessment with monitoring and tracking of the pain and a consistent and constant evaluation of the effectiveness of the medication is crucial. Age, gender, weight, muscle mass, state of disease, state of mind, and pain experienced are all things to consider when initiating and maintaining a pain management program.

In this chapter, I will explain the medications generally used to control pain. This will serve as your guide to the classes of drugs prescribed. Please do not construe the following information as medical advice. Only your physician can make the determination of which medications are best for your particular type of pain.

The actual approach to prescribing pain control medication is (and should be) very systematic. The guidelines are well established. Several resources are used in determining what is used and when. The main organizations that have established these guidelines are: The World Health Organization, The American Pain Society, and the Agency for Health Care Policy and Research (AHCPR). The two latter organizations have publications which serve as clinical guides on pharmacological, physical, and psychosocial ways to manage cancer pain. The World Health Organization established the widely accepted 3-step analgesic ladder in 1990.

These clinical guides are for professional use, but because they are easy to read and understand, I recommend that every person who has a pain issue obtain them. They are free of charge or sold at cost and will prove to be a valuable asset for you when consulting with your physician (see Appendix 7).

The 3-step analgesic ladder is the starting point for determining the medication regimen. The ladder gives a wide scope of options that may be used within a class of drugs.

Step 1 For mild to moderate pain.
> Use the simplest dosage of a non-opioid drug with or without the use of an adjuvant (explained below): aspirin, acetaminophen, or nonsteroidal anti-inflammatory drug (unless contraindicated).

Step 2 When pain persists or increases.
> Add an opioid.

Step 3 If pain continues or becomes moderate to severe.
> Increase the opioid potency or dose.
> Dosing should be on an around-the-clock schedule.

What is an Adjuvant?

Adjuvant therapy is treatment with substances that enhance the action of drugs. Some adjuvant drugs help to potentiate, that is, to increase the strength or activity of a drug. They are used in combination therapy. For instance, the use of a nonsteroidal anti-inflammatory drug (NSAID) is often included in combination with an opioid when pain becomes moderate and has failed to be controlled with analgesics such as aspirin, acetaminophen, or a nonsteroidal anti-inflammatory drug alone, like Motrin. The NSAID is the adjuvant therapy with the opioid.

On the 0-10 pain rating scale, mild to moderate pain would be from 2-5, with 2 being mild and 5 being moderate. In this range, we try to start with a non-opioid drug alone. Similarly, we don't automatically start with an opioid at level 5 and above until we have tried a non-opioid first.

0-10 Numeric Pain Intensity Scale

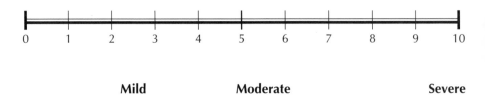

Mild   Moderate   Severe

Nonsteroidal Anti-Inflammatory Drugs - (Non-opioid Drugs) — aspirin, acetaminophen and nonsteroidal anti-inflammatory drugs (NSAIDS).

These drugs are used for mild to moderate pain. Side effects from these drugs can occur and they should be used with caution, as ulcers or bleeding tendency may develop at any time. Monitoring for toxicity is essential, especially if the patient is taking Coumadin, antidiabetic medications, Digoxin, or sulfa drugs. Also, many over-the-counter drugs already contain a high dosage of acetaminophen.

There is a ceiling, or maximum amount, in dosage that a person can take of these drugs. Overdosage can lead to toxicity and organ damage. The maximum recommended dose of acetaminophen is 4000 mg./day. Nonsteroidal anti-inflammatory drugs should be used with extreme caution by the elderly as well as by those who have a tendency towards ulcers, or have decreased hepatic function, renal failure, or bleeding tendencies.

NSAIDS - nonprescription

- acetaminophen - Lacks anti-inflamatory and antiplatelet activities of the other NSAIDS. Total allowable daily dose of acetaminophen is 4,000 mg./day.

- aspirin

- ibuprofen (Motrin, others)

Only one type of NSAID at a time should be given. Acetaminophen is the exception, and can be given with a different NSAID. The total daily doses need to be monitored to prevent side effects and toxicity.

NSAID - prescription (Sample list) Usual adult doses if body weight is greater than 50kg (110 lbs.).

- **Dolobid**   500 mg.   Every 12 hrs

- **Lodine**   200-400 mg.   Every 6-8 hrs

- **Orudis**   25-60 mg.   Every 6-8 hrs

- **Toradol**   10 mg.   Every 4-6 hrs
                                to a maximum of 40 mg./day
                                for short-term use only

- **Naprosyn** 250-275 mg.   Every 6-8 hrs

Reference adapted from AHCPR - *Management of Cancer Pain: Adults*, Quick Reference, 1994.[1]

Patients with thrombocytopenia (reduced blood platelets) should not take analgesics (nonsteroidal anti-inflammatory drugs), because of the risk of bleeding.

For example, patients receiving chemotherapy would not likely be given aspirin because of its effect on blood platelets (chemotherapy lowers the platelet count and results in the risk of bleeding). High doses of acetaminophen are associated with liver toxicity. Long-term use of these drugs is not recommended and so a move to the second step on the World Health Organization's 3-Step analgesic ladder would be appropriate when pain continues or increases.

Use of Opioids (Narcotics) for Pain Management

As we discussed earlier, many patients, families, and physicians are fearful of the use of narcotics in pain management. Yet this is the class of drugs that is the mainstay for relief of pain. The many regulations regarding prescription painkillers are meant to prevent abuse and addiction, yet addiction is very rare: 1 in 1,000-10,000 when these opioids are used to control pain. Each state medical board institutes its own policies and the problem is that there aren't any pain experts on these boards to help establish reasonable and ethical policies and guidelines concerning pain control.

The standards of practice and use of narcotics set forth in the guidelines established by the World Health Organization, the American Pain Society, and the Agency for Health Care Policy and Research are widely accepted in the medical community. However, there are still many physicians who either ignore the existence of these protocols or haven't taken the time to study them and integrate them into their practice. These standards can and should be adopted by state medical boards so that the correct pain medications in the proper dosages are available to all patients who need them.

Again, every patient is unique and requires a physician to establish the appropriate regimen. The following is an overview of the opioids used to control pain. The principles cited here are for educational purposes only. Dosages may vary and readers are advised to verify the accuracy and appropriateness of all dosages with their medical professional.

Narcotic

A narcotic (opioid) is derived from opium or is produced synthetically. Opioids act by binding to receptor sites in the central nervous system. They can induce euphoria, mood changes, mental clouding, and sleep, and can depress respirations and the cough reflex. Most opioids cause side effects of constipation and/or nausea. Side effects are treatable by 1) decreasing the dose and/or the interval between doses and 2) changing the opioid. Anyone receiving an opioid should be on a bowel regimen aimed at softening the stool and they can promote evacuation with a mild laxative (unless contraindicated).

Narcotic Agonist

An agonist is a drug that has a specific cellular affinity that produces a specific response of analgesia (pain relief) at the spinal level. The agonist is absorbed from the gastrointestinal tract (there are opiate receptor sites in the bowel). This is why there is a side effect of constipation. The motility, or movement, of the bowel slows down, impeding the movement of waste through the bowel. This is correctable with the bowel regimen as stated earlier.

The narcotic agonist is the class of drug that is used to control pain that is moderate to severe. Codeine, Darvocet-N, Demerol APAP, fentanyl citrate, hydrocodone, and morphine sulfate are just some of the 45-plus drugs your doctor can choose from.

Narcotic Antagonist

The antagonist drug has an opposite action to that of the agonist, or competes for the same receptor site. The narcotic antagonist reverses the effect of the agonist, causing immediate withdrawal symptoms: nausea, vomiting, sweating, rapid heart beat, tremors, seizures. It is given to reverse the effects of the agonist when overdose has occurred. Overdosing is not common and, in my years of experience, I have never had a patient who experienced a problem of overdose. The most common narcotic antagonists used to reverse respiratory depression (a sign of overdose) are: Narcan (naloxone hydrochloride) and Trexan (naltrexone hydrochloride).

How Narcotics Are Usually Prescribed

The primary indicator for the use of a narcotic is the level of pain a patient is experiencing. A narcotic regimen is indicated for persistent moderate to severe pain (level 5-10 on a 0-10 pain scale). Usually, a nonsteroidal anti-inflammatory drug is given first. If there is no relief, then a weak opioid is added, like codeine. Below are some examples of the weak opioids. The usual starting doses are also indicated.

Combination Opioid and NSAID Preparations

- **Codeine** — with aspirin or acetaminophen.
  Starting dose: 60 mg. every 3-4 hours.

- **Hydrocodone** — Morphine derivative that is similar to codeine.
  Trade names: Hycodan, Robidone, Vicodin (codeine with acetaminophen), Lorcet, Lortab, and others.
  Starting dose: 10 mg. every 3-4- hours.

- **Oxycodone** — synthetic derivative of opium with actions similar to morphine. More effective for acute pain than for long-standing pain.
  Trade names: Percocet-5, Percodan, Roxicet, Roxicodone.
  Starting dose: 10 mg. every 3-4 hours.

Reference adapted from AHCPR - *Management of Cancer Pain: Adults*, Quick Reference, 1994.[1]

For those people who are allergic to codeine, a synthetic form of codeine can be used, which is Vicodin (see above). There may still be cross-sensitivity, but it is not usual. The effectiveness of these and all other drugs is measured by using the pain scale that you have seen in the previous chapter. If pain continues, your doctor can go in one of three directions: 1) increase the dose of your current medication, 2) change the drug to a different weak opioid, or 3) go with a higher level narcotic at a lower dose. If pain is at a level 5 or above and is persistent, then a lower starting dose of a stronger narcotic is indicated.

Morphine Sulfate

The most frequently prescribed narcotic is morphine sulfate. This is the drug of choice for long-standing cancer pain. There is no ceiling to the amount which is prescribed because effectiveness is measured by the amount of relief. There have been doses given of up to 10,000 mg. (10 grams) a day. The usual starting dose is 10-30 mg., every 4 hours.

Morphine sulfate is a natural opiate used for severe or chronic pain. Variably absorbed from the gastrointestinal tract, its peak action is reached in one hour if taken by mouth, 20-60 minutes by rectum, 50-90 minutes by subcutaneous injection, and 20 minutes if given intravenously. The duration of pain relief lasts up to seven hours when taken in the immediate-release form.

There is an extended-release form of morphine sulfate, which is MS Contin. This extended release is intended for use every 8-12 hours. It comes in 15 mg., 30 mg., 60 mg., 100 mg., and now 200 mg. tablets. The 200 mg. tablets are for use in the opioid tolerant patients who require 400 mg. or more of daily doses. The extended-release tablets should never be crushed, broken, or chewed. This would result in overdose characterized by respiratory depression (slow respirations), somnolence, stupor progressing to coma, cold and clammy skin, low blood pressure, and sometimes a slow heart rate.

Immediate-Release Morphine

Immediate-release morphine can be administered by mouth (tablet or solution), subcutaneous injection or infusion, intramuscular injections, intravenous infusion with a pump that also has a patient-controlled bolus button for breakthrough pain (see next page), or by rectal suppository. It also can be placed in the stoma of a patient who has a colostomy.

It is advisable, according to the product information guide, to start with the immediate-release form. Titration of the medication (adjusting the dosage to achieve the desired effect)is more reliable and immediate. Titration is continued until the desired effective relief is established. Once the relief has been sustained, then a switch to the extended form can be effected. There are conversion tables in the product guides provided by the manufacturer: The Purdue Frederick Company, Norwalk, CT.

A pain scale rating should be done at peak onset of the drug, which is one hour after administration by mouth, and again at the hour the next dose is due. If a person is ambulatory and eating, we don't worry about respiratory depression too much because it is usually not clinically significant in a person who is up and around. With the bedbound, more debilitated person, we would monitor more closely and, yes, we would check respirations by counting them in one minute's time. If respirations decrease to 10 or below (12-18 is normal), then the patient would have to be monitored at regular intervals, and the physician should be notified.

Now, if pain is not controlled within 24 hours on the low dose, then the dose may be increased by 50-100 percent. If pain persists and the patient was receiving morphine sulfate at 30 mg. every 8 hours (extended release), the dose could be increased to 45 mg. and up to 60 mg., to be taken every 8 hours. A smaller dose increase would be used for the elderly patient (usually starting at 25 percent of the dose we would give a younger person), and we would work our way up as needed.

Duragesic Patch

Another very popular narcotic is the Duragesic Patch (fentanyl citrate). This is a medication that comes in the convenient form of a transdermal patch, meaning that the medication is delivered via absorption through the skin. The patch has to be changed every 72 hours. Careful consideration should be given as to who should use this drug. It is not recommended for someone who is elderly or debilitated because clearance of the drug (the removal of a substance from the blood via the kidneys) is usually prolonged and this can cause a health threat for a weakened person. The starting dose should not be higher than 25 mcg./hr (micrograms per hour). Decreased respirations may occur at any time, and residual medication of up to 50 percent is present in blood serum 17 hours after removal of the patch. I have found that patients have better pain control management with morphine sulfate since the Duragesic Patch peak action time is 12-24 hours, whereas the peak action time of morphine sulfate is 60 minutes.

Breakthrough Pain

Sometimes a patient may experience breakthrough pain. This is pain that develops several hours before the next dose of medication is due. The standing dose of medication may not have to be increased. In the case of breakthrough pain, the physician may order a fraction of the dose of what is being taken as the standing dose. Note how often breakthrough pain occurs and do a pain-scale rating. If the pain is mild (2-4 on the pain scale) then a nonsteroidal anti-inflammatory drug may be all that is needed. If the pain scale is 5 or above, then a supplemental narcotic dose may be needed. You would need to call your physician.

If breakthrough pain occurs more than four times a day, your physician would have to consider increasing the standing dose of the opioid drug. It is better to increase the dose and keep the same hourly spread than to increase the dose and extend the hourly spread. For instance: if you are taking 30 mg. of morphine sulfate every 8 hours and pain persists or is not relieved, then it is better to increase the dose to 45-60 mg. but keep it at every 8 hours, rather than extending the time to every 12 hours. Once it is given, the breakthrough medication would be discontinued until further evaluation of pain relief. The medication used for breakthrough pain should be the same class of drug as what is being prescribed as the standing medication. For example, fentanyl citrate and morphine sulfate are both morphine narcotic agonist drugs.

Roxanol is frequently used for breakthrough pain, as is Dilaudid. Roxanol is liquid morphine (immediate release) oral solution. It comes in 10 mg./2.5 ML, 20 mg./5 ML, 30 mg./1.5 ML. Roxanol has a maximum analgesic effect occurring in 60 minutes.

Dilaudid (hydromorphone) is more potent than morphine and can be used as the standard medication for pain or as a supplement for breakthrough pain. Dilaudid is 8-10 times more potent than morphine. There is also less nausea and vomiting associated with this drug. It has a more rapid onset with a shorter duration of action: peak onset is 15-30 minutes, the duration of the drug lasts 4-5 hours. The usual starting dose is 1 to 4 mg., every 4-6 hours. If given rectally, 3 mg. every 4-6 hours. A conversion chart is available from the manufacturer, Knoll Pharmaceutical Company, New Jersey.

Conversion charts are used when the medication is changed from one form of a narcotic to another. It's called equianalgesic dosing. For instance, if you are taking 60 mg. of morphine sulfate, the equivalent dose of Dilaudid would be 7.5 mg., and of codeine, 200 mg. These conversion charts are necessary if the physician wants to switch from one narcotic regimen to another, while keeping the same dose effect for pain relief.

The Calculation of Breakthrough Medication

To calculate the dose needed for breakthrough pain medication, the physician would total the amount of milligrams you are taking in a 24 hour period. Let's say you are taking 30 milligrams of morphine sulfate every 8 hours. The total amount is 90 milligrams over a 24 hour period. This number is divided by 6 (one sixth of the total dose). The amount of milligrams used for the breakthrough pain would be 15 mg. of morphine sulfate every 2-4 hours as long as breakthrough pain exists, while maintaining the dose of 30 mg. every 8 hours. Again, if breakthrough pain occurs more than 4 times a day, the physician should consider changing the dose of the standard medication you are receiving.

I have seen very good pain control with morphine sulfate (trade names: Astramorph PF, Duramorph, MSIR, MS Contin, Roxanol), as well as with Dilaudid and, to a lesser degree, the duragesic patch. I have never seen respiratory depression in any of my 400 plus patients. Side effects were always controlled and most patients remained alert and were able to have improved ability to function.

Delivery

The routes by which these medications are delivered are many, as you have seen. The route is most often determined by the patient's level of function, physical condition, and choice. In most cases, pain can be well controlled by taking the medication by mouth.

Injections are not recommended for long-term pain management because of discomfort and anxiety associated with them. Also, there is always the possibility that the medication intended for intramuscular administration winds up in a blood vessel by accident, resulting in overdosage.

The intravenous route is very effective for pain control, but this route is recommended for the bedbound patient who cannot easily swallow pills and who has severe pain. With intravenous administration monitoring for respiratory depression is routine. However, the dosages required to relieve pain are relatively small: 2 mg./hour. Incremental dosing is done gradually, if needed, and patients often tolerate this route very well.

The dosing guidelines for both non-opiate and opiotic analgesics established by the World Health Organization include:

- By mouth — this is the preferred route and should be used whenever possible. Alternative routes include rectal, transdermal (through the skin), or continuous intravenous infusion.

- Around the clock — this means that medication should be administered at regularly scheduled times on a 24 hour basis. The elderly and seriously compromised patients need diligent monitoring for the first 24-48 hours for side effects. For the elderly, breakthrough pain medication is usually 5-15 percent of the total daily dose and can be given every 1-2 hours for pain.

- By the Ladder — The World Health Organization has established a 3-step protocol (explained earlier) on when non-opioids and opioids should be administered.

The Use of Antidepressants and Anticonvulsants as Adjuvant Therapy

As explained earlier, adjuvant therapy enhances the action of other drugs. Antidepressants and anticonvulsants are used to treat neuropathic pain, which is characterized as inflammation of the peripheral nerves, resulting in shooting and burning pain. This form of pain can be caused by tumor compression causing inflammatory response, or by nerve degeneration. This pain is usually chronic and the most problematic. The exact mechanism of action of these drugs is not known, but it is felt that tricyclic antidepressants help by interferring with the re-uptake of serotonin and norepinephrine (neurotransmitters).

Antidepressants optimize the effects of the opioids by decreasing hypersensitivity to the pain response. Elavil and Paxil are drugs commonly used. They not only help to control pain, but are effective for mood elevation. The disadvantage is that patients can experience what is called anticholinergic side effects: dry mouth, urinary retention, and constipation. Side effects can be controlled by drug and non-drug methods.

Anticonvulsant drugs most often used to treat neuropathic pain are Clonazepam and Phenytoin (dilantin).

It is important for you to know that antidepressants are not being given to treat depression when you have pain — they are only being used to affect the pain response. Also, it takes several weeks for serum levels to reach an adequate level; you may not feel the full effect until that time.

In summary, adjuvant therapy may include:

- a nonsteroidal anti-inflammatory: some common drugs in this class are Aleve, Advil, Motrin, Aspirin, Toradol, Feldene, Naprosyn, Orudis, Lodine.

- the use of a narcotic: morphine sulfate, Duragesic Patch (fentanyl citrate), Dilaudid, and others.

- a tricyclic antidepressant: Elavil (amitriptyline), Pamelor (nontriptyline); or an anticonvulsant: Dilantin (phenytoin), Clonidine (catapres), to name a few.

The Use of Steroids to Control Pain

Steroids have a multifunctional use in the treatment of pain. Corticosteroids have an anti-inflammatory effect as well as a mood elevating effect that serves to promote an overall feeling of well-being. These drugs may be used as adjuvant therapy with opioids. Another advantageous effect is that appetite is stimulated. Long-term use may result in hyperglycemia (high blood sugar level) and dysphoria — a change in mood.

Since there is a high incidence of spinal cord compression relating to lung cancer, corticosteriods are useful in relieving edema (swelling) associated with pressure on the nerves.

Reference adapted from AHCPR - *Management of Cancer Pain: Adults,* Quick Reference, 1994.[1]

Some Precautions for Patients Taking Steroids

- People taking steroids should be cautioned not to take aspirin or medications containing aspirin.

- Insomnia may occur.

- Always take with food to avoid gastric irritation.

For Patients with Bone Metastases

There is a relatively new product (1993) being used to control pain in those patients who have documented metastases to the bone. Metastron (strontium-89 chloride injection) is an aqueous solution of strontium-89 chloride for intravenous injection. It often is used in combination with radiation therapy. Strontium-89 is a radioisotope that localizes to the bone, relieving pain associated with bone metastases. According to the product literature, a single dose of Metastron provides pain relief for up to six months, often reducing or eliminating the need for dose escalation of narcotic analgesics. Pain relief occurs on an average of 7-20 days following administration.

The use of Metastron in persons with seriously compromised bone marrow is not recommended. Depression of bone marrow activity is expected following administration, lowering the white blood cells and platelet counts. Bone marrow activity recovers within six months of treatment. This drug is meant only for those patients who have documented metastases to the bone. Ask your radiation oncologist if Metastron is appropriate for you.

A Story about Pain and Medication

At this point, I'd like to tell you about a patient of mine who didn't get the care she needed, and why. It had been two months since I last saw this patient. Recently I had received a call from her husband saying she was in the hospital. He was lamenting the fact that she was admitted for the purpose of giving her intravenous fluids because of dehydration. "Now they want to do gallbladder surgery and also put in a Greenfield filter for a blood clot," he told me. I asked if I could go with him to the hospital.

It was 7:30 p.m. when we arrived. We were appalled at what we saw. She was dying. She was in agonal breathing. She couldn't speak and her face grimaced torturously in pain (they had discontinued the Duragesic Patch she was on). Her body lay helpless in an uncomfortable position with her legs extended out through the bars of the side rails of her bed. She looked at me with wide-eyed terror.

My first thought was: where is her nurse? Just then, this cocky miss walked in and rushed over to the beeping IV machine. She never looked at her patient, or said a word to either her husband or me. After she had finished her mechanical task, she fully intended on leaving the room without so much as a glance towards the patient, until I stopped her. Blocking her path, I asked if the patient was getting anything for pain. She said the patient wasn't in pain, and left the room.

I tried to elicit a response from the patient. She was aware and was trying to communicate, but couldn't. I took a large pad and wrote out the numbers one to ten. Holding the pad so she could see it, I asked her to help me assign a number to her pain. I pointed to each number and asked her to blink twice when I came to the number. She blinked twice at 9. I repeated, "You're having a level 9 pain?" She blinked again.

Calling the nurse back in, I asked what was ordered for pain. "Morphine 2 mg. an hour p.r.n.," she said. "When was the last time she got her medication?" I asked. "She didn't get any because she's not in pain, she's moving around," she said. I told her the patient was in severe pain and to get the house doctor to give it now. When the house resident physician arrived, 15 minutes later, he administered the morphine IV push. I complained that the p.r.n. order needed to be changed to around the clock because no one was assessing her for pain, and the pain level warranted ATC (around-the-clock) management. I asked him to call her primary doctor for me.

While I was waiting, I watched for the signs of relief. I told her she had just been given the pain medication and that she would feel better in a little while. I repositioned her in the bed and held one hand while her husband held the other. I asked if she wanted a priest. It took all her strength to emphatically groan out a "yes."

I went out to find the nurse again. My contempt and anger grew by the minute. The phone rang in the room. It was her doctor. "Doctor, would you please change the order for morphine to be given ATC? No one is assessing her pain." I told him, "She is at a level 9. She can't verbally communicate, she's in agonal breathing, her extremities are blue, and she's pooling" (blood pools to the extremities in the hours before death). The doctor was concerned with acidosis (a complicated condition referring to the acid/base balance in the body). I firmly said, "what is more important, the acidosis or the extreme pain?" He changed the order for the morphine to be given every hour.

She remained awake and quieted down to a more peaceful rest. The priest arrived and anointed her with the last rights of her faith. Prayers were said aloud over the sounds of her agonal breathing.

I estimated she had four to six hours left. I tried calling different agencies to procure a special duty nurse who could stay the night. I didn't want her to be alone. I couldn't find one. The thought occurred to me to stay. But I was very tired and it was late. She could be like this all night. I knew she was getting her medication, and she had seen the priest. I talked to her about trying not to be fearful, that nothing bad was going to happen to her, that God loved her. I told her to think of her parents, who were waiting for her. "Think of only good things," I said.

We left. I called the hospital the next morning and was told she died during the night. A hospital is no place to die. She was spared the surgery, but was denied the dignity of dying at home.

Can you plainly see what was wrong here?

- The hospital staff never notified her husband of the change for the worse in her condition (she had been sitting up in the morning and had asked for a paper).

- The nurse never assessed her pain, nor did she take care of her patient's need for mouth care, repositioning, compassionate touching, or reassurance.

- The nurse never notified the doctor of the change in her condition.

- They failed to provide for pastoral care, until I asked for it.

- They were going to operate on a woman who had only hours left to live.

Never assume that because your loved one is in the hospital that he or she will be well cared for. You have to ask questions and make demands. She was in the wrong place at the wrong time. She did become pain-free and saw the priest — two accomplishments of notable importance. They have to count as triumphs. With your loved one, please be sure to:

- Ask what medications have been ordered, and at what intervals.

- Ask when your loved one last received his or her pain medication.

- Do your own pain scale rating with your loved one.

- Report the results to the staff.

- Ask if the order is p.r.n. (as needed) or around-the- clock. Remember the protocol is "around-the-clock."

- If it is p.r.n. and the pain rating is 5 or above, ask to speak to the physician.

- Ask the physician to change the order to around-the- clock.

Moral of the Story

Patients can and do receive better care at home. If your loved one is admitted to a hospital, this should not automatically be an event that signals relief. You have to be watchful that care is being given and your loved one's needs are attended to.

Hospitals and staff generally are not equipped to handle the special needs of the dying. People who are facing the last stages of death require a good deal of comfort care (to be discussed in Chapter Eleven). This requires time and an understanding of the person's psychological needs, and even more so if the patient is unable to speak. A nurse who has 12-15 patients simply cannot devote the necessary time to a dying patient. An uneaten dinner is whisked away without consideration of whether or not the patient was able to reach his dinner tray. Patients frequently lie in their own excrement because staffing is limited and a forgotten problem can be left for the next shift.

The general staff at hospitals does not have a real working knowledge of pain management. Excuses are used to disguise the fact that assessments are not routinely done. There is simply no real patient advocacy going on, so you shouldn't be too relieved when someone you love is admitted to the hospital. They may not be getting what they need and deserve.

The protocols for pain management are clear and concise. There are many people who are knowledgeable, but more who are not. The resources available are too many to mention. I have provided you with some of them in Appendix 7. They are all free and easy to obtain.

Conclusion

There are so many variables, factors, choices, demands, and concerns. Now you have the knowledge you need to maintain your loved one in comfort. The "opponents" I spoke of earlier in the Continuum of Pain model are those family members and/or medical professionals who are non-facilitators, who block your requests for pain management. After reading this chapter, you can converse on an equal level with these opponents. You can begin to take the path away from pain, and I assure you that if you follow it, it will protect you or your loved one from the depression, anxiety, and powerlessness that results from pain.

Let me reemphasize one important point. If your primary physician and/or oncologist is not knowledgeable in or sensitive to pain management, change to one who is — QUICKLY!

I have armed you with the information needed to challenge a prescribed course of treatment in an intelligent and rational manner. In many instances, you will know more than the physician you are debating with. Remember, you are either the patient or the patient's advocate. Also remember that the doctor may have his or her own agenda:

- Dying patients are often considered "write-offs." The doctor may feel the battle is over and nothing more can be done.

- Pain goes largely unassessed in medical situations.

- "Pain is normal" is used as a defense when the physician has inadequate knowledge in prescribing a narcotic regimen.

- "Time is money," and pain management takes time. Some physicians don't want to spend dollar time on a penny's worth of symptom control.

- "Let's look for bigger things to do." Often the dying are subjected to needless procedures or surgeries that highlight the physician's area of expertise and at the same time bring in added revenue. The "write-off" becomes the "add-on."

The general public does not know a great deal about medicine. You're not expected to know. However, you should know when you are being "taken." You may sense it, but are probably too forgiving and respectful to come to the conclusion that indifferent actions may be deliberate.

Praise the gods if you have a physician who is understanding, sensitive, and knowledgeable; one who puts the needs of you and your loved one above the worth of a co-payment. They are out there. Do your best to find one who is right and just. You will see him or her walking in the halls of honorable medicine.

Let me leave you with one last thought, best expressed by the World Health Organization: "Nothing would have a greater impact on cancer pain throughout the world than to put into effect the currently available knowledge about pain treatment. Helping cancer patients obtain relief from their pain is the concern of many health professionals worldwide, irrespective of country of origin and of existing health care infrastructure. The WHO (World Health Organization) encourages health professionals to understand the system that is used to make morphine and other opioids available to the patients who need them. This knowledge can make professionals more effective in identfying and removing barriers to opioid availability and can help them provide more effective pain treatment" (World Health Organization. Cancer Pain Release, 1994).

*   *   *   *   *

I think a fitting end to our discussion on relieving pain is an introduction to the inspirational power of philosophy. Philosophy can help in our search for the meaning of life and the importance of the individual. Our interest here is not in the interpretative value of philosophy, but rather in its comfort value. You'll see that whatever religious beliefs you have are probably not contradictory to the values and judgements of the great thinkers of the past.

This is where we have a chance to examine our feelings

about where we stand in the context of person to person, person to nature, person to the universe, and person to the realm of the beyond.

Come with me now, and I will take you for A Rest in the Field of the Philosophs.

Chapter Eight
A Rest in the Field of the Philosophs

Strive to continue to be such as philosophy wished to make thee. Remember the Gods, and help men. Short is life.

Marcus Aurelius Antoninus

S hort is life...how true for all of us. And because it is true, there is no better time than now to find hope for the soul. You will hear from some of the greatest philosophers of all time — master teachers of life, self, and soul. Their words are alive and relevant today, having endured over two thousand years. That is why I have chosen to take you to the Field of the Philosophs, a secret place of mystical beauty and enlightenment. The Philosophs will give you what you need...what we all need.

"As a child is born or comes into life by leaving the womb, so the soul may in leaving the body pass into another existence which is perfect."

This chapter is for all of you, regardless of your religion, culture, state of mind, or state of health. Together we will seek the meaning of life and our purpose while we live it. What we discover may change your priorities and shift your life in the direction of peace, tranquility, and hope. For as Marcus Aurelius once wrote,

"How plain does it appear that there is not another condition of life so well suited for philosophizing as this in which thou now happenest to be."

All of us have developed our own views that have contributed to our sense of self. We have, in effect, developed our own philosophies. We go through life with a preconceived notion that our philosophy is the true one. We often are not open to the views of others because they threaten the stability of our being. We are more comfortable living in an environment of personally lived experience rather than in an environment in which we can question possibilities. But is our way of thinking the only way? Is our truth the only truth?

Philosophy is the discipline that uses logic, aesthetics, and metaphysics to pursue wisdom, values, and understanding. The great thinkers of ancient times reach out to us today to challenge our understanding of truth, virtue, death, mortality, immortality of the soul, and our place in the universe. We are at the perfect juncture in our journey to explore the possibilities of what truth is. You may find that the questions that lay dormant in your mind will be brought forward in consciousness and enlightenment. You may very well find peace in what the ancient philosophers have said. Their words are not merely idle sayings, but rather they are thoughts and conclusions grounded in wisdom and logic that have survived as truths for centuries.

I am not a scholar of philosophy. I read it to be inspired, enlightened, comforted, and challenged. Philosophy has rearranged my former steadfast convictions into an exciting world of possibilities that I deem more probable than not. Philosophy does not contradict religious beliefs. It is complimentary to beliefs both in the divine and in nature. Is there one ultimate question? No, there are many. What is virtue? Why are we born? What is good? Does God watch over the world? What becomes of us after death? Is there a soul?

You are not one isolated being. You are indeed part of the whole creation that has purpose, meaning, and destiny. As such, you also have purpose, meaning, and destiny. You are not just Michael or Mary who has cancer. You are part of your parents, their parents, and so forth. We are all connected by the material of what is seen and unseen. Open your mind to the possibilities. Try to see yourself within the greater context of being part of the whole. There is still time to discover that philosophy has much to offer you. It can help you understand that which you question, that which is meaningful to you. It can help validate your existence by offering the conclusion that we are part of one universal intelligible whole: an ever-changing universe that holds within it ever-changing matter that is eternal. I want you to listen and find what is meaningful for you.

Come now as we Rest in the Field of the Philosophs. We will

use imagery to get there.

I can see there are legions of people with us now, as we move along the path away from pain. The path makes a gentle turn to the right. As we approach its end, it is now almost dark, but we see the most beautiful clearing. Huge pine trees surrounding the field stand closely side by side, as if in a majestic ceremonial stance. We have the feeling that we are in a special place. A pungent crisp scent of pine fills the night air. The sun has set, and the sky has a color of midnight blue, illuminated by a moonlight we have never seen before. We acknowledge one another with a knowing smile as we intuitively know why we are here — to experience something special. We rest and we wait. Thoughts of our past come to mind. We wonder if we have lived a good life. We wonder about the nature of our being. There is more. We know it.

The night takes on an unusual stillness. There, in one moment, a bright white flash appears behind us as wind and fury causes us all to look back. Unable to see through the flash of light, we feel we're moving, yet we are still together sitting as we were. We didn't move, **it** is coming to us! Muffled voices soon give way to clear speech. We are in a time and place not our own. It's daytime and though we can see those around us, we are unseen and unnoticed by the small group that has gathered in front of us. An older man is the center of attention as the younger men listen to his words with great interest.

Meno raises a question to Socrates:

> **Meno:** *And how are you going to search for something, Socrates, when you have no idea whatsoever what it is? What kind of unknown somewhat will you propose as the object of your search? And if you are lucky enough to come across it, how will you know it is that unknown somewhat?*
>
> **Socrates:** *They say the human soul is immortal: at one moment it comes to an end, what is called dying, at another it comes to rebirth, but it is never subject to*

annihilation...and so, since the soul is immortal and has been born many times, and has seen everything there is, both here and in Hades, there is nothing it has not learned. It is no wonder, then, that it has the capacity to recollect all that it formerly knew about virtue and so forth. All nature is akin: the soul has learned all things. There is no reason, then, why by recollecting one single thing — having learned it, as men say — it should not be enabled to find out everything else, provided the inquiry be conducted in a resolute and tenacious manner. Enquiry and learning are entirely recollection.

We know who Socrates is. We are in the year 399 B.C. amidst the glory of Athens, which prides itself on its influential thinkers. Socrates has spent his whole life here in poverty, for he would never take money for teaching matters of the soul, virtue, or courage. He is the wisest of all men yet claims to know nothing. However, there is a pall in the city and a sense of impending doom, because Socrates, now seventy years of age, is about to become a martyr for philosophy. A sadness falls upon us, we who are unseen yet aware that this man who held truth above all else would soon be executed for allegedly corrupting the youth of Athens.

The light of day is muted by an incoming fog that descends upon us like a curtain. There is a powerful control here, but for some unknown reason we remain unafraid. After moments of anticipation, the fog dissipates at once in all directions and we find ourselves in a torch-lit prison cell. We are here to witness not only the death of Socrates, but to learn from him the knowledge that would nourish our souls.

As silent bystanders, we see Socrates communing with his ardent friends who have gathered in his cavernous cell. A dank smell permeates the echo of their words.

Socrates: *For I am quite ready to acknowledge, Simmias and Cebes, that I ought to be grieved at death, if I were not persuaded that I am going to other* *gods who are wise and good...And therefore I do not grieve as I might have done, for I have good hope that there is yet something remaining for the dead, and, as has been said of old, some far better thing for the good, than for the evil.*

Cebes: *Tell me Socrates, why is suicide held not to be right?*

Socrates: *I suppose that you wonder why, as most things which are evil may be accidentally good, this is to be the only exception (for may not death, too, be better than life in some cases?), and why, when a man is better dead, he is not permitted to be his own benefactor, but must wait for the hand of another...*

I admit the appearance of inconsistency, but there may not be any real inconsistency after all in this. There is a doctrine uttered in secret that man is a prisoner who has no right to open the door of his prison and run away; this is a great mystery which I do not quite understand. Yet I, too, believe that the gods are our guardians, and that we are a possession of theirs. Do you not agree?

Crito: *The attendant who is to give you the poison has been telling me that you are not to talk much, and he wants me to let you know this; for that by talking heat is increased, and this interferes with the action of the poison; those who excite themselves are sometimes obliged to drink the poison two or three times.*

Socrates: *Let him mind his own business and be prepared to give the poison two or three times, if necessary; that is all.*

Socrates continues talking with his friends Simmias and Cebes while others gathered there listen. We, ourselves are gathered around Socrates and it is as though he is speaking directly to us.

> **Socrates:** *Whether the souls of men after death are or are not in the world below, is a question which may be argued in this manner:*

Socrates now speaks about an ancient doctrine that says souls go from this world into another and come back again born of the dead. He goes on:

> *Then let us consider this question, not in relation to man only, but in relation to animals generally, and to plants, and to everything in which there is a generation, and the proof will be easier. Are not all things which have opposites generated out of their opposites? I mean such things as good and evil, just and unjust — and there are innumerable other opposites which are generated out of opposites. And I want to show you that this holds universally of all opposites; I mean to say, for example, that anything which becomes greater must become greater after being less.*

> **Cebes:** *True,...*

> **Socrates:** *Well, and is there not an opposite of life, as sleep is the opposite of waking?*

> **Cebes:** *True.*

> **Socrates:** *And what is that?*

> **Cebes:** *Death...*

> **Socrates:** *And revival, if there is such a thing, is the birth of the dead into the world of the living?*

> **Cebes:** *Quite true.*

Socrates goes on to tell us that there are two sorts of existences — the seen and the unseen. The soul is unchangeable as compared to the body, which is changeable. The soul is governed by the divine and the body is "subject or servant" to the soul.

Socrates: *That soul, I say, herself invisible, departs to the invisible world — to the divine and immortal and rational: thither arriving, she lives in bliss and is released from the error and folly of men, their fears and wild passions and all other human ills, and forever dwells, as they say of the initiated, in company with the gods. Is not this true, Cebes?*

Cebes: *Yes, beyond a doubt.*

After much discussion, those gathered (including Socrates) meditate on the arguments made regarding the soul's immortality, wisdom, and perfection. The group is trying to understand how Socrates can remain so calm at a time when death is so imminent.

Socrates: *Will you not allow that I have as much of the spirit of prophecy in me as the swans? For they, when they perceive that they must die, having sung all their life long, do then sing more than ever, rejoicing in the thought that they are about to go away to the God whose ministers they are. But men, because they are themselves afraid of death, slanderously affirm of the swans that they sing a lament at last...And I, too, believing myself to be the consecrated servant of the same God, and the fellow servant of the swans, and thinking that I have received from my master gifts of prophecy which are not inferior to theirs, would not go out of life less merrily than the swans.*

Again, after some time of further discussing the soul, Socrates goes off to the bath chamber. Upon returning, his jailor laments at having to give Socrates the cup of poison to drink and asks his forgiveness, for no one so noble or honorable had been in his prison before. Then bursting into tears, he turns away and goes out.

> **Socrates:** *How charming the man is; since I have been in prison he has always been coming to see me, and at times he would talk to me, and was as good as could be to me, and now see how generously he sorrows for me. But we must do as he says, Crito; let the cup be brought, if the poison is prepared: If not, let the attendant prepare some.*

Socrates holds the cup of poison and drinks without hesitation. His friends wail out their cries. We don't want to witness this but the images are ever present, as is the damp smell of the prison.

> **Socrates:** *What is this strange outcry? I sent away the women mainly in order that they might not offend in this way, for I have heard that a man should die in peace. Be quiet then, and have patience...Crito, I owe a cock to Asclepius; will you remember to pay the debt?*

> **Crito:** *The debt shall be paid; is there anything else?*
> (There is no answer.)

Socrates lays dead, lifeless and silent. The cries of those around him mourn not only for the loss of a friend, but for the thought of never hearing his prophetic wisdom again. For he was a connection to the eternal truth, a guide who brought the soul's recollection of knowledge to their consciousness and to ours. He had spent his 70 years on earth in search of the meaning of mankind's existence. He had "corrupted" the youth by teaching virtue and values. He lives on in the Field of the Philosophs, bringing his message of hope to those who fear life ends in death. He tells us to care for our souls, to seek beauty and wisdom in life. He aspired to universal truths: the unchangeable and unseen essence of beauty and good. The meaning of our existence lies not in the material, for that is purely for the benefit of the body, the changeable and the seen. For Socrates, the meaning of existence is in knowing thyself: to dignify the soul by always seeking truth.

The vision slowly dissipates in a white fog as small, bright flashes appear through the haze. Again a voice is heard. The fragrant scent of pine reassures us we have not been taken elsewhere. The voice we hear is that of a narrator, who is telling us about Plato.

We see him plainly now, seated on a large rock. His voice is rich with tenderness yet he speaks with authority. We have the feeling this man knows who we are, yet his identity is unknown to us. His white tunic bears a Roman look of distinction, far greater than that of an ordinary Roman citizen. We are taken by his pride and graciousness.

This man speaks to us of Plato, the student and friend of Socrates. He tells us that it is only through Plato that we have come to know Socrates because Socrates had never written anything down. He tells us:

> Plato's dialogues recount the teachings and philosophy of Socrates, as well as Plato's own ideas and thoughts. In the dialogues, Plato expands beyond the concepts of the immortal soul to include a metaphysical foundation of reality: reality, in true form, is perfect, unchanging and eternal. And, according to Plato, this true reality is found in "Forms" or "Ideas."

> These Forms or Ideas are universal and exist beyond what we perceive as the real world. All that we see and "know" in this world is a distorted reflection of reality that is subject to time, change, and deterioration. The true form of reality exists in an unchangeable, eternal sense. Plato says that only the soul, which is immortal and unchangeable, can come into the knowledge and contact of the Forms

themselves. What are these Forms? There is the Form of Good, for example, that is eternal and exists as a pure form of what good is.

The narrator points to one person and says: "You may think good means doing something kind for someone else." Pointing to another, he says, "And you may think good means the absence of hurting someone."

"Good" is open to your interpretation. However, Plato says there is one definition of good — the Form of the Good, which is like the sun: an unchanging eternal reality. Good leads to justice, which in turn leads to harmony of the soul. Happiness is harmony in a person who has cultivated a just life. Plato expanded on what Socrates had thought about the self to include an ordered system moved by a creator: "A one over many." Existence for the self is always a pursuit of value.

The man seated on the rock pauses as he looks carefully at us gathered around him. A voice from the crowd cries out, "Who are you?" The man says, "It is I...Marcus Aurelius." Spontaneous applause rings out and Marcus, his arms out, attempts to lull us into silence. We are acquainted with his words from our journey thus far, and we wait to hear what more he has to say:

Yes, I am Marcus Aurelius, born in the year 121 A.D. During my life, I was a Roman emperor and a philosopher. They say I was the last distinguished representative of Stoic philosophy. Like Socrates and Plato, I too believe in the permanence of the soul and the universe. I would like you to listen for a moment as I read from my personal meditations. These are my practical expressions by which I have lived; a kind of moral compass to set one's path.

This then remains: Remember to retire into this little territory of thy own, and, above all, do not distract or strain thyself, but be free, and look at things as a man, as a human being, as a citizen, as a mortal.

I am composed of the formal and the material; and neither of them will perish into nonexistence, as neither of them came into existence out of nonexistence. Every part of me then will be reduced by change into some part of the universe, and that again will change with another part of the universe, and so on forever.

Nothing happens to any man which he is not formed by nature to bear.

Accustom thyself to attend carefully to what is said by another, and as much as it is possible, be in the speaker's mind. That which is not good for the swarm, neither is it good for the bee.

Just as it is with the members in those bodies which are united in one, so it is with rational beings which exist separate, for they have been constituted for one cooperation. And the perception of this will be more apparent to thee, if thou often sayest to thyself that I am a member of the system of rational beings.

That which has grown from the earth to the earth, but that which has sprung from heavenly seed, back to the heavenly realms returns.

Look within. Within is the fountain of good, and it will ever bubble up, if thou wilt ever dig.

Everything exists for some end, a horse, a vine. Why dost thou wonder? Even the sun will say, I am for some purpose, and the rest of the gods will say the same. For what purpose then art thou? To enjoy pleasure? See if common sense allows this.

He who fears death either fears the loss of sensation or
a different kind of sensation. But if thou shalt have no
sensation, neither wilt thou feel any harm; and if thou
shalt acquire another kind of sensation, thou wilt be a
different kind of living being, and thou wilt not cease
to live.

Marcus Aurelius slowly closes his book of meditations and looks out over the people. His expression is compassionate. We sense his desire that we understand what he has read.

The mood is reverent and respectful. We know he has come to help us find meaning in our existence. The mortal presence of Marcus gradually transforms into a translucent image that finally fades completely from sight. The rock which was barely noticeable before is a dominant reminder of what we have just seen and heard. We are all taken up in the moment of this extraordinary occurrence.

What did these men of the ages come to tell us? The human soul is immortal. The body is subject to the laws of the divine, which govern the universe. The soul cannot be annihilated. All learning is entirely recollection because the soul, being immortal, has knowledge of all things. Death is the release of the soul from the body: a separation from hinderance. The soul has an affinity with justice, goodness, and truth.

The message is that we should strive to care for our soul in this earthly life. When we act in a manner that is just, we enrich our soul. Socrates had said no man knowingly does wrong because we know intuitively that doing wrong would harm our soul.

What else have we learned? We live in a universe that is highly ordered. Nothing occurs by accident. Everything has a purpose and a meaning that is designed to teach us lessons. This is perhaps why, even in ancient times, the act of suicide was considered forbidden. The general inference is that we are not permitted to "quit" the tasks assigned to us in this life, even if that task requires great suffering, whether it be physical or emotional. There seems to be some retribution to be paid if we leave life before we are ordained to leave.

According to Socrates, everything is generated out of its opposite: heat, cold; the greater, the lesser; and so forth. It is a process of continual change and transformation that never ends. Socrates makes the same analogy for life and death, that each is generated out of the other.

"Then there is a new way in which we arrive at the inference that the living come from the dead, just as the dead come from the living; and if this is true, then the souls of the dead must be in some place out of which they come again," says Cebes.

Socrates replies, "If generation were in a straight line only, and there were no compensation or circle in nature, no turn or return into another, then you know that all things would at last have the same form and pass into the same state, and there would be no more generation of them."

We see this same reference from Marcus Aurelius many centuries later when he writes:

That which has grown from the earth to the earth, but that which has sprung from heavenly seed, back to the heavenly realms returns.

Marcus Aurelius tells us to live by nature and according to nature. Nothing happens that is beyond our capacity to bear. Be free by living outside the opinions of others. Hold on to your own truths, for they will bring you tranquility. He feels that if we look deep enough within ourselves, we will find only goodness. Further he says:

Take pleasure in one thing and rest in it, in passing from one social act to another social act, thinking of God.

As a child is born or comes into life by leaving the

*womb, so the soul may on leaving the body pass into
another existence which is perfect.*

Our mission in life, it appears, is to learn and grow in
knowledge and goodness. As mortals, we have choices in
every situation presented to us. We all know intuitively how
to choose a course of action that will benefit us the most. But
are we looking towards a primal benefit? That is, one that
will satisfy our basic instincts for pleasure. Or can we choose
a course that probably requires some sacrifice that will
ultimately lead to an intangible yet pleasurable satisfaction
of the soul? I believe that is what we are here to learn. Can
we make the right choices? Can we forgive those who we feel
have transgressed against us? It seems that we must do so if
we are to move on to a higher spiritual dimension. The
mission of our life on earth is to learn love, forgiveness, and
understanding.

Regarding an afterlife, if the soul is immortal and we do not
cease to live, as the philosophers have said, then it stands to
reason that they did believe in an afterlife.

Roman Afterlife

Cicero was born 106 B.C. He was schooled in philosophy at
the Academy founded by Plato, and became a legal consul in
Rome, where he advocated for a constitutional government, in
direct conflict with Julius Caesar's dictatorship. Caesar had
offered political positions to Cicero, who refused numerous
times. After the assassination of Caesar, Cicero wrote a
dialogue in defense of Brutus.

Cicero often referred to Scipio, born 185 B.C., in his many
essays and other writings. Scipio himself was an orator and
political activist in Roman politics many years before Cicero's
time. Cicero's major work, *On the Republic* (51 B.C.), portrays
Scipio as the principal speaker. The last book of *On the
Republic* — *Scipio's Dream* is the creation of Cicero's
imagination but is based on Plato's analysis of the immortal
destiny of the soul. Here then, are excerpts from Scipio's

Dream in which he saw his deceased grandfather and father.
Reprinted by permission of the publishers and the Loeb Classical Library from *CICERO: DE RE PUBLICA, VOLUME XVI*, translated by Clinton W. Keyes, Cambridge, Mass.: Harvard University Press, 1928.

Upon recognizing him I shuddered in terror, but he said: "Courage Scipio, have no fear, but imprint my words upon your memory."

Though I was then thoroughly terrified, more by the thought of treachery among my own kinsmen than by the fear of death, nevertheless I asked him whether he and my father Paulus and the others whom we think of as dead, were really still alive.

"Surely all those are alive," he said, "who have escaped from the bondage of the body as from a prison; but that life of yours, which men so call, is really death. Do you not see your father Paulus approaching you?"

When I saw him I poured forth a flood of tears, but he embraced and kissed me, and forbade me to weep. As soon as I had restrained my grief and was able to speak, I cried out: "O best and most blameless of fathers, since that is life, as I learn from Africanus, why should I remain longer on earth? Why not hasten thither to you?"

"Not so," he replied, "for unless that God, whose temple is everything that you see, has freed you from the prison of the body, you cannot gain entrance there. For man was given life that he might inhabit that sphere called Earth, which you see in the centre of this temple; and he has been given a soul out of those eternal fires which you call stars and planets, which, being round and globular bodies animated by divine intelligences, circle about in their fixed orbits with marvelous speed. Wherefore you, Publius, and all good men, must leave

that soul in the custody of the body, and must not abandon human life except at the behest of him by whom it was given you, lest you appear to have shirked the duty imposed upon man by God. But, Scipio, imitate your grandfather here; imitate me, your father; love, justice and duty, which are indeed strictly due to parents and kinsmen, but most of all to the fatherland. Such a life is the road to the skies, to that gathering of those who have completed their earthly lives and been relieved of the body, and who live in yonder place which you now see" (it was the circle of light which blazed most brightly among the other fires), "and which you on earth, borrowing a Greek term, call the Milky Circle."

"Strive on indeed, and be sure that it is not you that is mortal, but only your body. For that man whom your outward form reveals is not yourself; the spirit is the true self, not that physical figure which can be pointed out by the finger. Know, then, that you are a god, if a god is that which lives, feels, remembers, and foresees, and which rules, governs, and moves the body over which it is set, just as the supreme God, above us rules this universe. And just as the eternal God moves the universe, which is partly mortal, so an immortal spirit moves the frail body."

He departed and I awoke from my sleep.

As we rest in the field of the Philosophs, it is fitting that we contemplate all that we have seen and heard. We have the opportunity to examine our inner beliefs while at the same time remaining open to the teachings of the ages. How wonderful it is to look at humankind as one intelligible whole, irrespective of religion or ethnic background. We all share the same concerns and uncertainties. We all share the same desires for happiness and peace. We are one kind, moving according to the order of the universe.

The words of the philosophers who lived centuries ago sound like the words we would hear today. Scipio's apprehension at having to remain on earth until the ordained time is like any other person's, given the situation. We haven't changed over the ages. Technology of course has changed, but not the human condition. We are still subject to disease, politics, wars, and mortality — but of the body only. We can and will transcend mortal difficulties. This is our purpose.

This life is equivalent to a nanosecond when measured within the context of eternity. Separation of any kind is only temporary. Like a leaf that falls from the tree into a flowing stream, the others soon follow to eventually join in union at the beginning of a great expanse. The portal of hope is endless and limitless. Trust in the recollection of your soul that you will go on to eventually join in union with all those you have loved and who have come before you.

And this is why our creator has given us the capacity to hope. It is hope that drives us upward towards the light. It is hope that allows us to think in terms of possibilities. Hope is the portal through which truth and knowledge can be attained. For the sake of courage, for all that you wish to see and learn, I ask you now to climb the hills of hope.

Chapter Nine

Now Climb the Hills of Hope

*All things are implicated with one another, and the
bond is holy; and there is hardly anything unconnected
with any other thing...For there is one universe made
up of all things, and one God who pervades all things,
and one substance, and one law...Be thou erect, or
be made erect.*

Marcus Aurelius Antoninus

What exactly is hope? Can it be adequately defined? To me, hope is a desire for fulfillment. We hope for many different things. We hope for a better life, a better job, for health and happiness. The list is endless. So where do we begin to break all these hopes down to several manageable gifts of inspiration? To have hope, you need to be inspired and I consider inspiration to be a gift. Hope is a gift. The ability to hope transcends the scientific realm of empirical evidence and explanation. We often hope for things that seem impossible to achieve or obtain. Yet, these impossible events or happenings occur every day. It is hope that moves the human spirit beyond its own self-limiting boundaries. It is hope that moves the universe towards change and transformation. It is hope that makes miracles happen.

Is it realistic to hope for a miracle? While miracles don't occur in abundance or to everyone, they do occur. Often, medical practitioners cannot explain the shrinkage of tumors or the complete abatement of cancerous lesions after traditional treatment has failed. There simply is no scientific explanation for such things. There is no explanation for the 4.4 percent of people who walk out of Calvary Hospital, each year, cancer-free. Similar statistics were quoted by Memorial Sloan-Kettering, another world-renowned cancer treatment hospital. There is no harm in hoping for a miracle. In too many cases, it is truly the last resort.

In the last chapter you read about hope for the soul. I would like you to refer back to that chapter whenever you become disheartened. Our bodies are given to us for only a short time. Sooner or later we are all going to have to submit to its frailty. But the frailty is in the body only, not the soul. Socrates' view of the body was that it is a nuisance:

> *For the body is a source of endless trouble to us by reason of the mere requirement of food; and also is liable to diseases which overtake and impede us in the search for truth; and by filling us so full of loves, and lusts, and fears, and fancies, and idols, and every sort of folly, prevents our ever having, as people say, so much as a thought.*

Never before has there been such a concerted global effort in the fight against cancer. Every day we read about some drug, gene therapy, or treatment that holds promise for control, if not eradication, of cancer. Thousands of scientists around the world are working feverishly to bring you hope. Billions of dollars are spent on clinical trials, cancer prevention, and cancer control measures. This is a global issue. It is not limited to the United States. Cancer was once a word whispered in secret, little talked about and not addressed. Today, it is shouted out as an enemy of humanity and humanity is fighting back.

Global Cancer Incidence

Worldwide, there were 52 million deaths in 1996. Of those, 6 million people died of cancer. Lung cancer claimed 989,000 lives and there were an estimated 1.32 million new cases. Deaths from other cancers were: stomach, 776,000; colorectal, 495,000; liver, 386,000; and breast cancer, 376,000. There were almost three times as many deaths from lung cancer as there were from breast cancer. Smoking causes one in seven cancer deaths worldwide. At least 15 percent of all cancers are a consequence of chronic infectious disease, the most important being hepatitis B and C viruses (liver cancer), the human papilloma virus (cervical cancer), and the helicobacter pylori bacterium (stomach cancer).

In 1996 there were an estimated 17.9 million persons

worldwide with cancer who survived up to 5 years after diagnosis.

Cancer Incidence in America

The year 2000 estimates for new cancer cases were over 1.2 million. Approximately 11 million cases have been diagnosed since 1990. The good news is that some of the approximately 8 million Americans alive today who have a cancer history can be considered cured.

Progress Against Cancer

In 1996, the American Cancer Society, the National Cancer Institute, and the Centers for Disease Control and Prevention reported that for the first time in history we had turned the corner in our fight against cancer. New data showed that in the early 1990s, overall death rates from cancer began to decline as a result of intensified efforts to prevent, detect, and treat cancer.

Data published in the March 15, 1998 issue of the American Cancer Society's oncology journal, *Cancer*, show that cancer incidence rates are decreasing for all cancer sites and the death rates from cancer continue to decrease.

A press release from the National Cancer Institute on September 30, 1998 stated:

- Five-year survival rate for children with cancer improved from 65 percent in the early 1980s to 74 percent in the early 1990s.

- The five-year survival rate for all cancers improved from 51 percent in the 1980s to almost 60 percent in the early 1990s.

- Two million women who had breast cancer are alive today.

- One million men are survivors of prostate cancer.

Hope on the Horizon

Every day, we read about some new and innovative drug, treatment protocol, or clinical trial. Research is being conducted at maximum speed and new discoveries are being announced in quick succession. However, it takes years, sometimes 10 years, before a promising drug modality arrives in prescription form. There are particular quandaries associated with testing animals to assess a drug's effect on people. What often works in the animal can prove ineffective in humans.

Researchers have previously focused on killing cancer cells with cytotoxic drugs and radiation, which have their own inherent side effects and complications. Now scientists are discovering possible ways of disarming the cancer cells on their own DNA level through genetic warfare. Molecular diagnostics, molecular medicine, and gene therapy are leading the scientific community towards new approaches in research. The conventional approach of understanding the way in which a cancer cell grows, mutates, and destroys other cells (carcinogenesis) has shifted to a cancer cell's genetic process.

Normal cells become cancer cells by transformations that take place at the gene level. Genes make proteins that govern cell multiplication. One protein is called epidermal growth factor (EGF). When a retrovirus gets into a cell, it takes control of the cell's own EGF gene. The EGF gene becomes an oncogene (a cancer causing gene) due to the production of large amounts of the EGF protein, which cause epidermal cells to grow in an uncontrolled fashion. Bladder cancer in humans, for example, is caused by a single mutation of a gene.

Mutations that occur in a normal cell are often the result of exposure to natural and synthetic compounds that are carcinogenic. Between 70 to 80 percent of cancers in humans are related to chemical and environmental factors.

Induction is the first stage in the multistage carcinogenesis. It occurs when exposure to chemicals, radiation, viruses, and smoking produces modifications in the normal cell which makes it precancerous. It appears that the genetic composition of the host (a person) is important in cancer induction. Promotion and conversion are the last two stages and may take up to twenty years to develop. In other words, someone might be exposed to a carcinogen, like smoking, as a young adult but they may not develop symptoms of cancer until years later.

Gene Therapy

Cancer is a disease of the genes. Earlier, I mentioned that genes make proteins that govern a cell's growth. Gene therapy is aimed at regulating the genes and their specific protein synthesis. (Proteins are responsible for much of the structure of body cells and are related to physiological functions.) Gene therapy manipulates genetic material inside the cancer cells or material inside the immune cells. For example, genetically engineered viruses have been used in gene therapy to replace damaged genes with healthy genes.

Breast Cancer Breakthrough

Molecular analysis is an up-and-coming scientific trend. There are many companies involved in molecular diagnostics. ONCOR is one such company. In 1990, ONCOR became the first company to receive FDA approval to market a gene-based cancer testing system for the diagnosis of leukemia and lymphoma. Most recently, the company received FDA approval to market the first gene-based test for assessing the risk of recurrence and death associated with lymph node-negative, invasive breast cancer.

What is HER-2/neu? HER-2 /neu is one of 100,000 genes found in every cell of the body. This gene has the potential of becoming an oncogene (cancer causing gene). In some breast cancers, the HER-2/neu gene is present in extra copies. Thus, the protein HER-2 is produced in excess, causing an excessive proliferation of cancer cells.

INFORM HER-2/neu Detection System   This detection system by ONCOR is a Fluorescence In Situ Hybridization (FISH) DNA probe assay that determines the qualitative presence of HER-2/neu amplification (extra copies of the gene). It is used as a prognostic indicator.

If you have had or currently have breast cancer and want to know your HER-2/neu status, your physician can request the test to be performed on archival tumor material. This test does not replace tests currently in use, but it is used as a strong predictor of risk for recurrence of breast cancer. For information, call 1-800-77-ONCOR.

Genetic Vaccine Helps Immune System

Researchers Dr. H. Kim Lyerly and Eli Gilboa from Duke University's Center for Genetic and Cellular Therapies in Durham, NC, are studying the safety and effectiveness of a new immune system therapy called a genetic vaccine.

The vaccine creates a precise attack on a particular abnormal cell growth. The vaccine utilizes the patient's own cancer cell's genetic makeup. Researchers say this treatment is safe for the elderly or for people who have a weakened immune system. This does not prevent cancer, but may stop the spread of cancer or recurrence. (On Health, 10/21/98)

Is a Cure on the Horizon?

It seems that the scientific community is getting close to finding not only new answers but new potentially effective means of at least prolonging life for the cancer patient. The new field of biotechnology has grown tremendously and there are now over 200 new drugs relating to cancer.

Antiangiogenesis Drugs

Harvard researcher Judah Folkman has used two drugs, Angiostatin and Endostatin, to stop tumors from creating their own blood supply, essentially starving cancer cells. Dr.

Folkman has spent thirty years researching cancer cells. He has determined that the growth and spread of cancer cells are dependent on their ability to form blood vessels. The vessels then carry nutrients to the cells enabling them to grow.

Clinical trials for Angiostatin and Endostatin began in the fall of 1999. Meanwhile, there are clinical trials currently in operation for other antiangiogenesis drugs. A new antiangiogenesis agent, called TNP-470, has been developed. This synthetic chemical is being used to slow the growth of kidney cancer. Researchers report that side effects are mild and there is a high incidence of prolonged progression-free survival. They deem this to be very encouraging. For information call 1-800-4-CANCER.

New Drug Therapies for Breast Cancer

Tamoxifen has been used for twenty years in the treatment of advanced breast cancer. It acts by slowing or inhibiting the growth of breast cancer cells. Now the drug is believed to prevent the disease in those who are cancer-free, but who are at risk, and it has been approved by the FDA to be used as a preventative drug. Tamoxifen is highly toxic and has a life-threatening side effect, namely thrombosis (blood clots), so it is important to remain under close medical supervision during Tamoxifen therapy.

Herceptin — FDA approved September 25, 1998. This drug is for the treatment of women whose breast cancer has spread beyond the breast and lymph nodes. Herceptin targets cancer cells that overproduce the protein HER-2. This overproduction occurs in about 30 percent of breast cancer patients. Herceptin blocks the growth-promoting attribute of HER-2 and may help the immune system recognize and attack the breast cancer cells.

Herceptin was tested on 691 women with metastatic breast cancer that carried the extra copies of the HER-2/neu gene. When results of treatment with standard chemotherapy alone versus chemotherapy plus Herceptin were compared, it was found that tumors shrank at least 50 percent in half the women getting chemotherapy with Herceptin, compared with one-third of women receiving chemotherapy alone.

Raloxifene is a drug used for the prevention of breast cancer. In clinical trials, Raloxifene (also used for osteoporosis) has been shown to cut the risk of breast cancer by 70 percent without causing endometrial cancer. For more information, call 1-800-4 CANCER for the latest or current studies that you might be able to participate in.

Xeloda — FDA approved April, 1998. Approval for this drug was based on a trial of 43 patients whose cancer no longer responded to conventional treatment. In that group, Xeloda appeared to help shrink tumors in 25 percent of the patients. In a larger study involving 162 patients, tumors shrank in 20 percent of the patients. (Centerwatch.com, September 13, 1998).

The FDA warns that Xeloda is neither a cure nor does it help everyone, but it showed such promise that they approved it early in the testing process.

Lung Cancer Breakthrough

A study published in the September, 1998 issue of *Nature Medicine* concerned a preliminary trial using gene therapy to treat lung cancer. The trial involved nine men with advanced lung cancer. They all had a mutated copy of the tumor suppresser gene, P53. Researchers injected healthy copies of the gene into the patient's cancerous lung tissue once a day for five days.

The lung tumors treated with P53 solution stopped growing in three patients and regressed in another three. The significance of this trial indicates that gene therapy may be effective in halting cancer progression.

The researchers were led by Dr. Jack A. Roth of the University of Texas MD Anderson Cancer Center. (*Nature Medicine* 1996; 2: 985-991)

Drug Therapy for Lung Cancer

Gemzar — FDA approved August, 1998. This drug is indicated in combination with Cisplatin (a chemotherapeutic drug) for the first-line treatment of patients with inoperable, locally advanced, or metastatic non-small cell lung cancer. It is also indicated as first-line treatment for patients with locally advanced adenocarcinoma of the pancreas. Gemzar is indicated for patients previously treated with 5-FU, a chemotherapeutic agent.

Prostate Cancer Breakthrough

The breakthrough is a new test that is a spin-off of the widely used Prostate Specific Antigen (PSA) blood test. The new test is called **free** PSA, or PSA II. The prostate gland produces a glycoprotein by the cells of the ductal epithelium of the prostate, and is present in the blood serum of all males. This specific protein is called prostate-specific antigen (PSA). The PSA is increased in prostate cancer and is also increased when there is an enlargement of the prostate gland, called benign prostate hypertrophy (BPH). Enlargement of the prostate is a normal occurrence with increased age of men over 50 years. A normal PSA level is 0 - 4 ng/ml. However, a PSA reading above 2.0 ng/ml in men with a normal sized prostate, should raise concern for prostate cancer. Typically, a PSA reading of 10.0 ng/ml would indicate the need for a biopsy of the prostate gland to confirm the presence of cancer. In March, 1998, a new blood test was approved by the FDA. This test is the PSA II or free PSA. The free PSA is a measure of how much prostate-specific antigen is circulating alone in the blood and how much is bound together with other proteins. The free PSA test is performed when there are PSA levels between 4 and 10. If the free PSA is 25 percent or less, there is a 95 percent cancer detection rate through biopsy. This means that cancer can be detected earlier by using the free PSA test, when the PSA test alone gives a result of 4 - 10 ng/ml. For more information on Prostate cancer, detection, and treatment, go to **cancerorg.com**. (American Cancer Society), or **Prostrcision.com**. (Radiotherapy clinics of Georgia).

According to the American Cancer Society, men should begin screening for prostate cancer at age 50. However, men in high risk groups — especially those who have a family history of prostate cancer — should begin at age 45. There is curative treatment for prostate cancer if it is detected early. The 1998 estimate is 89 percent for five years or longer survival rate.

This year, the American Cancer Society has earmarked approximately $7.5 million dollars for prostate cancer research. There are several new areas of research for prostate cancer.

- Development of a new technique to examine lymph nodes of men with prostate cancer. This could have an impact on staging (identifying the level of cancer involvement).

- Development of a vaccine-like treatment that would trigger an attack on cancer cells.

- The University of Pennsylvania reported in their internet cancer information service, *Oncolink*, that a certain herpes gene may help fight prostate cancer. A phase I study examined 18 patients who had local recurrence of prostate cancer following radiation. The herpes gene activates a normally inactive antiviral drug, Ganciclovir. When the herpes gene was successfully transferred into the prostate cancer cells, the Ganciclovir was activated, killing the cancer cells. The PSA levels decreased significantly in 3 of the 18 patients. One person showed no sign of cancer after a biopsy was performed.

Other New Tests and Drugs

Reuters Health Information (an online information service), reported that a pencil-sized probe for cervical cancer may be available soon. The device was tested in 15,000 patients at London's Whittington Hospital. The device, called a polar probe, emits wavelengths of light and electrical impulses. The head of the probe detects the return signals and compares it with the computer to search for cancer or precancerous tissue. The reported sensitivity is 97.6 percent and a 91.1 percent detection rate of carcinoma of the cervix.

There is now reason to be hopeful when there is **metastasis to the bone**. Often, patients with advanced lung, breast, and prostate cancer develop this secondary cancerous invasion to the bone. A study reported in the *New England Medical Journal* in August, 1998, revealed promising prevention with the use of the drug Clodronate. There were 302 women with breast cancer who were involved in the study. Half were given the drug for two years along with standard treatment of chemotherapy, hormonal therapy, and surgery. The other half were not given the drug, but received the same standard treatment. New tumors were detected in 42 women who did not receive the drug. Only 21 of the women who took the Clodronate had developed distant tumors. There are other drugs on the market now which are similar — Pamidronate and Alendronate. Ask your oncologist if any of these drugs are appropriate for you.

New Cancer Drug Being Tested; Hope for colon cancer, head and neck cancer. The drug called IMC-C225, was developed by Dr. John Mendelsohn of Memorial Sloan-Kettering Cancer Center in New York City. The drug was first tested in 1999 on a 30 year-old with metastic colon cancer. Cancer had spread to her liver and abdomen, and was not responding to chemotherapy treatment. The cancer was advancing and when it became clear that chemotherapy would not halt the multiple tumor growth, IMC-C225 was tried for the first time, in a human. Used in combination with a chemotherapeutic drug, Camptosar, her tumors shrank 80%. The remaining tumors were surgically removed. Today, she is considered cancer-free. No doubt, there will be many clinical trials in the coming year involving this remarkable drug, IMC-C225. One such clinical trial will involve head and neck cancer.   And, there is always the possibility that scientists like Dr. John Mendelsohn will find new applications for treating many more forms of cancer.

A New Technological Advancement

The vast amount of research currently being done around the world has also resulted in the hardware technology breakthroughs that we are seeing in use today. I am speaking of 3D computer technology. This breakthrough is absolutely revolutionary and offers special hope for people with **brain tumors**. BrainLab is a German-based company responsible for the development of **NOVALIS**, a shaped beam surgery system for brain tumors. The significance of this technology is that the beam is perfectly conformed to the malignant tumor, and therefore does not harm healthy tissue. The procedure is completed in only a few hours and has fewer complications than the traditional invasive surgery. There is only one cancer center in the United States that has this technology. **NOVALIS** is being used to treat patients at UCLA's Johnson Cancer Center. For information call (310)825-9775 or find the website at **www.ucla.edu.**

The new advances described on the previous pages are just some of the breakthroughs that have been made in the quest for a cure for cancer. There are so many resources available to you. Your computer is the best link in finding them. If you don't have a computer, ask a friend or family member to help you search the **INTERNET.** There are thousands of links to information. Your local American Cancer Care or Cancer Society can also give you much of the information you need.

About Clinical Trials

Oftentimes, a clinical trial may be a person's "last" hope. (I never believe in "last" hopes, for there is the faith factor that you cannot ignore, but I will talk about this in the next chapter.)

Clinical trials are tests of new drugs that scientists have been working on for years. In the beginning, a research scientist tests these chemicals, proteins, or compounds on animals. They submit their data to the FDA, which then grants permission for clinical trial if the data shows promise. There are three phases to a clinical trial. The first, Phase I, is designed to make sure the experimental drug is safe to use in humans. A small group of 20-100 people are given the drug on a voluntary basis. About 70 percent of experimental drugs pass this first phase of testing.

Phase II involves testing the drug for effectiveness. There are two groups involved. One group is given the drug while the other group gets a placebo, an inactive substance that is harmless. Sometimes testing involves a double-blind study. This means that neither the patient nor the investigators know which group is getting the experimental drug or the placebo. The experimental drug is identified by a code.

Phase III involves testing hundreds or thousands of patients. These are randomized and blinded trials. About 90 percent of the drugs tested complete this phase.

Funding for clinical trials comes from many different sources but usually it is provided by the Federal government and/or pharmaceutical companies. The FDA requires all patients to sign an informed consent before entering a clinical trial. The National Cancer Institute also sponsors and monitors many clinical trials. (See Appendix for Chapter Nine for resources.)

If you are considering participating in a clinical trial, you should find out if it is necessary to stop your traditional therapy while participating in the clinical trial. You would have to seriously consider the benefits and risks involved in doing so, if this is the case. Also, remember that if you are in a Phase II study that requires a control group — the group that receives the placebo — you have a 50/50 chance of not getting the experimental drug. Talk with your oncologist about your options for a clinical trial. You shouldn't have to make the decision on your own.

*   *   *   *   *

The American Cancer Society has been responsible for many groundbreaking discoveries in cancer research. The Society has invested over 2 billion dollars in grants and research projects throughout the country. The efforts of the Society have resulted in a cure for childhood leukemia, the discovery of a chemotherapeutic agent 5-FU, which is now widely used to treat many kinds of cancer, monoclonal antibody therapy to treat lymphoma and other cancers (pioneered by Dr. Ronald Levy), genetic engineering; the discovery of suppresser genes which suppress formation of tumors, and many more discoveries which have led to better understanding of and treatment for this disease.

Our hope belongs to the scientific pioneers who use an ordered approach consistent with their scientific methodology. It is their discoveries, made within this framework, that will hold up to validation, as opposed to claims made by word of mouth of a "new discovery" of an ancient botanical that "cures cancer." Hope often makes us run in scattered directions and caution is needed to keep from going down a path that leads nowhere.

Alternative Medicine and Cancer

Why do people choose alternative medicine over traditional Western medicine? Do they think exotic herbs, extracts, potions, and secret formulas hold the key to a cure that would only be balked at by empirical scientists?

The answer to the first question is a mystery. We do not know why alternative or complementary therapies are being sought after so actively, yet 425 million visits in the United States were made to alternative medicine practitioners in 1990. A study reported in *Journal of the American Medical Association* in May, 1998 surveyed 1035 people in the United States. The researcher, John A. Astin, Ph.D. concluded that those seeking alternative medicine did so because they felt that it was more closely linked to their own beliefs, philosophy, and values regarding their health.

In answer to the second question, yes, many people do believe that these ancient herbs and extracts hold the key to a promise of a cure. And this may be a very dangerous assumption. The danger lies in rushing to conclusions and foregoing proven methods that are backed by clinical trials with the most rigid standards. These ancient formulations of natural origin are not bound by any regulation and someone who wants desperately to live will seek out anything that sounds like hope, especially if touted by a hope-master — a clinician who has something to gain.

What we now call alternative medicine and therapies have been used for centuries throughout the world. And there are so many therapies which are beneficial: therapeutic touch, biofeedback, acupuncture, acupressure, aroma therapy, massage therapy, even magnet therapy. However, it is the unconventional "medicine" that needs close attention, especially as it relates to cancer treatment.

People have stopped their chemotherapy because they were told it is poison, and have grasped at the wrong brass ring. The price paid for such decisions may be more than what people would be willing to pay if they knew the consequences. It takes time to test these unconventional medicines and only legitimate clinical testing can bear the weight of a claim.

That is why the Federal Government allocated 20 million dollars in 1998 to fund studies of alternative treatments at eleven newly created research centers. In 1992, Congress established the National Center for Complimentary and Alternative Medicine (NCCAM) within the Office of the Director of the National Institutes of Health.

This national effort hopes to provide a means to comprehensively evaluate alternative medicine practices. Other government agencies which collaborate with the NCCAM are the World Health Organization, Food and Drug Administration, and the Centers for Disease Control, among others. The NCCAM has established a clearinghouse to provide the public with information and accurate coverage of current activities. (See Appendix for Chapter Nine).

Cancer patients, beware of claims made by alternative medicine practitioners who say they have a product that cures or regresses cancer. The American Cancer Society has position statements on 714-X, Essiac, and antineoplastins stating there is no scientific evidence that the use of these treatments has any effect on cancer.

The Society urges people with cancer to remain in the care of qualified doctors who use proven treatment methods. I agree.

Remember, not all herbal remedies are harmless. The dietary supplement industry is not regulated by the FDA and they are not required to provide information on ingredients, safety, purity, or efficacy. Some of these remedies can cause life-threatening side effects, like blood clots.

PC-SPES, a popular over-the-counter remedy for prostate cancer, contains potent estrogenic activity and may produce clinically significant adverse side effects, especially if a patient is already receiving hormonal therapy. (*New England Journal of Medicine*, 1998; 339: 785-91). Benign sounding product names and their corresponding general description of use "to maintain prostate health" or "leg vein health" can be deadly to an unsuspecting consumer without the advice and consent of a physician.

Your hope is in the drug research of qualified scientists who use clinical trials to establish product safety, purity, and efficacy. Your hope is in the government agencies and cancer organizations that have your health and protection as their priority.

There are so many advances being made now. There is every reason to believe that there will be a cure for cancer. Already, chemotherapeutic drugs can cure most cases of childhood leukemia. There are currently millions of breast cancer survivors. We are already in the new frontier of gene therapy and combination drugs. There is hope for humanity, and as long as hope exists, the possibility of a cure exists.

We have journeyed through the hope for the soul and the hope for the body. And somewhere in between is another dimension to human experience: the dimension of divine intervention. Unlike science, this phenomenon cannot be easily validated. On the contrary, it is believed and accepted on the basis of faith alone, which has no defining criteria for acceptance. Faith, like hope, is another portal to possibilities through divine intervention.

This connection to the divine comes to us in the forms of answered prayers, visions, and miracles. It is God's way of easing our mind, healing our body, touching our soul, or simply conveying the message that we are loved and He is with us. While these gifts may not be experienced by everyone, they are no less significant for the whole. It is enough that they occur to some so that others will be inspired through faith.

I will take you now to the Mountain of Visions, where you will see the wonders of divine intervention.

Chapter Ten
To the Mountain of Visions

*Either the Gods have no power or they have power.
But if they have power, why dost thou not pray for
them to give thee the faculty of not fearing any of the
things which thou fearest...And who has told thee that
the Gods do not aid us even in the things which are in
our power? Begin, then, to pray for such things, and
thou wilt see.*

Marcus Aurelius Antoninus

We have traveled over much terrain in these past chapters. The terrain has been difficult, I know. We have also had moments of rest and peace. But if you feel there is something missing, you're right. We cannot talk about you as a person with an illness without helping you discover who you are as a person who has spiritual needs. While this is a subject that one usually finds within the quiet of one's soul, it often helps to see how others have connected to the spiritual side of life.

God loves you more than you or I could ever love anyone or anything. Yet we go through life often feeling alone or abandoned, unseen and unknown by the One who has created us. We wax and wane in our faith. It is good when life is good and poor when we are poor of soul. We need to know that we are loved. We need to know that our life has purpose. Why else are we here? In other words, we look for continued reassurance. We look for some sign of God's acknowledgment of us. We look for answered prayers, visions, and miracles.

We are heading to the Mountain of Visions, where you will see glorious signs of God's acknowledgments. I take you to the mountain because it is here where you can be assured that you are not forgotten. From here, the clouds and stars of the firmament can be seen without the distraction of chaotic life below. Look out from the mountain. I want you to see faith from its highest vantage point. I want you to see hope manifested in glory. I want you to see that the best is yet to come.

The gifts of answered prayers, visions, and miracles happen every day to ordinary people. You need not be a religious cleric or even a devout practitioner of your faith to experience divine intervention. These unexplained celestial gifts occur when we ask for help. It happens when we recognize that we cannot walk this way alone. It happens when we ask God for mercy in our plight. And sometimes, even asking a saint or a deceased relative to intercede can bring answers to our prayers. Sometimes, extraordinary things occur when you least expect them. For example, people have seen visions of a deceased loved one, usually after being distraught over their death. These experiences leave them comforted with a feeling that a nonverbal message was conveyed. The message from the other side is peace, happiness, and reassurance.

I am sure that at some point in everyone's life, a prayer is said to ask for help. And I am sure that there are those of you who feel your prayers were never answered. Tragedy can still loom in spite of having said our prayers. The answer may not be what we had asked for, but it may still be His answer. His answer may come in the form of courage or comfort. It may come in the form of a realization that we must submit to His will, for a greater purpose. Our confusion and frustration can sometimes lead us to despair and loss of faith. It is all a paradoxical mystery. A mystery we are not meant to understand. Only with the experience of hindsight can we see that if a certain thing had or hadn't happened years or months ago, we wouldn't be where we are today. All things happen for a purpose.

A prayer that was said long ago may be perceived as unanswered at the time. Only with the passing of time can you realize that it was indeed answered. Answers to prayers may be symbolic in nature. A prayer said to find a specific item may be answered by finding something you never knew you lost.

Ordinary people experience extraordinary things. No one person is any better or any more special than another. Why, then, do some people experience such extraordinary events as miracles, and others don't? I don't know. But I believe it is possible for everyone to experience some kind of divine intervention, even a miracle.

I'm an ordinary person who is probably average on the

"goodness scale." Yet, I have experienced many extraordinary things throughout my life. I do have a strong faith, but many people are probably more devout than me. I keep my faith between myself and God. I deserve no more consideration than anyone else. Yet, my experiences have been so profound that I never question the fact that God is here and is listening. He may send an angel, a saint, or another intermediary or He may come and provide help Himself. The reality is that prayers are answered and gifts are given to anyone who asks.

Rest now, as you read about real people who have had prayers answered, seen visions, and experienced miracles. The following stories were contributed by people who are aware of what this book is about. It is their gift to you. I have also included some of my own experiences. We want you to know that you are not alone, and there is hope in the truth that we are all connected, all loved by God, and that you will find eternal peace and happiness beyond what is humanly comprehensible.

The Ring

When I was a child about 8 years old, I lived with two sisters and a brother who collectively referred to me as "the brat." Of course, it was just a case of being misunderstood! My mother was my protector and so naturally I ran to her with every little tattle tale I could tell. Being the baby in the family, I had diplomatic immunity from harm. But my sisters did not welcome the idea of sharing a room with me.

My sister Mary is three years older than me. She was the neat one, always fastidious with her things, and she knew exactly where everything was. It was nearly impossible to touch anything of hers without Mary knowing about it. This is what made for an exciting challenge when I took her things, because heaven help me if I got caught. It required nearly perfect dexterity and precision to put something back the way she had it. Sometimes I got caught, which led to screaming cat fights, a real disruption for the family.

On Mary's eleventh birthday, my Aunt Josie gave her a beautiful "diamond" ring. I suppose it was glass, but to me it was the prettiest ring I had ever seen. Everyone was gathered around as Mary showed each one of us her treasure. I'm sure that when she got to me, she probably said something like, "Now don't touch this."

The ring was my biggest temptation. I was in a moral dilemma. I rationalized that I would not be stealing the ring, only borrowing it. I would have it back in her ring box, underneath the two folded shirts in her top right drawer that same day. So, I went ahead and borrowed it.

I was having such a good time at school that day, showing my friends and teachers the ring that Aunt Josie gave me! It was too big for my finger and I completely forgot about it as I played in the school's enormous playground. I felt very special that day…until I noticed that the ring was no longer on my finger!

That realization cut into my heart like a knife. Oh God! What was I going to do? Aunt Josie would never forgive me for losing her gift to Mary. Mary would scream and my mother would think that I was a thief and not love me anymore. I would be disgraced. I was beside myself with fear.

I waited for everyone to leave the school. I searched the floors and hallways to no avail. The only other place it could have been was somewhere outside in the school's enormous playground. And then I remembered Aunt Josie telling me that if I ever lost anything, I should pray to Saint Anthony, but I had to promise him a rosary or money for the poor for helping me. Being poor myself, the only thing I could offer was the rosary.

Looking around to make sure no one was watching, I walked out onto the playground and immediately was humbled by the great expanse of green grass before me. I was as contrite as an 8-year-old could possibly be.

Convinced that there was no way to find the ring on my own, I got down on my knees, put my hands together, and looked to heaven. I told Saint Anthony what I had done. I made an apology and asked for his help. I also promised a rosary and said that I would always have faith for the rest of my life if he would only help me find the ring. Still on my knees, my gaze left heaven's direction with the intention of bowing my head. For some reason, I turned my head slowly to the left and then stopped. At first, I didn't see anything. Then, there in the grass, at the other end of the playground, maybe 50 yards away, was a bright flickering light that seemed to be calling to me. I stood up and without taking my eyes off this flickering light, I walked and then ran across the playground until I reached it. I bent down and picked up the shining object — — it was the ring! I couldn't believe it! It was so far away from where I was praying. He does hear my prayers! He does hear my prayers! I'm forgiven!

The real answer to that little girl's prayer was not finding the ring. That prayer changed my life and gave me faith. God and Saint Anthony have been with me ever since. To a child, that was a miracle. To an adult, it is an interesting story. To me it will always be a miracle.

There have been many other "little" divine interventions in my life. And there were a few that were miracles on a higher order.

"Saint Anthony, Help Me!"

When I was 22 years old, I was living at home with my parents, in the midst of planning my wedding, which was only 6 weeks away. Emotionally, I was still a child. I had clung to my parents all my life, something I am not ashamed to admit. I loved them very much. I wanted and needed to believe that they would live forever. Take me instead, I would pray when Mom or Dad was sick, for I felt I would die without them anyway. Those prayers were not answered.

One hot summer morning, I was awakened by my mother's voice calling out my father's name. "Jack, Jack." Again I heard, "Jack, Jack" in a pleading voice. I jumped out of bed and ran into my parents' room. There on the floor, my father was lying motionless. My mother couldn't move. She was in shock. She was a trained registered nurse and she was standing over him frozen. I heard my father exhale loudly. He didn't take another breath. I didn't know what to do. "Mom," I yelled, as if I could jolt her into action. "Give me the respirator!" I put the mouthpiece in his mouth hoping that would force air into his lungs. Nothing. I straddled him and started chest compressions. I had no idea about what I was doing. I was just imitating what I thought I saw once. Taking a breath, I then blew one deep breath of air into my father's mouth. Nothing, no response. Oh God, terror welled up inside of me. While my hands were still on his chest, I turned my head back and threw a sharp glance at the Saint Anthony statue on the dresser. In one desperate plea I yelled, "Saint Anthony, help me!" Turning back to my father, I compressed his chest three more times. After the third compression, he took in one gasp of air and opened his eyes. In that same instant, I felt an immensely holy presence next to me, and the room was filled with a haze that looked like a fine smoke suspended in stillness. My whole being was filled with an unearthly sense of ecstasy and peace. I stood up slowly in disbelief of what I was seeing and feeling. "Mom, look at the room," I said. "I see it, I see it," she responded. Not wanting to talk anymore, I stood perfectly still in the midst of this holiness. It lasted for about one minute. Then slowly, the holiness, ecstasy, and peace ebbed away gracefully and was gone. When it left, I felt sharply aware of its absence. The ecstasy and peace could not possibly be reimagined or re-created in a human sense. Nothing could compare to the joy that was given to me in that minute.

My father was conscious and was able to speak. I called 911 and shortly afterwards he was taken to the hospital. My mother rode with him in the ambulance while I stayed behind a few minutes to be in the room alone. Kneeling on the floor where my father had been lying and looking at the Saint Anthony statue, I began to sob over the gift we were given. "You were here, you were here," I cried. "I called and you came. I love you Saint Anthony. With all my heart, I love you."

My father had suffered a brain hemorrhage. The doctors

had given him a 50/50 chance of survival. Six weeks later, Daddy walked me down the aisle at my wedding. He survived another 16 years.

Sometimes we ask for something never really expecting it to come to pass. We may hope for it, but the request may be beyond what we deem possible. When our request is granted, we are truly touched by God.

The Sign

There is one last story from my own life that I feel I must tell you. It's about my mother. I adored my mother. We were blessed to have such a close bond. Perhaps it was because I was born with a hole in my heart and medical setbacks have a way of drawing loved ones closer together. My mother was a nurse who worked long hours and never complained of her hardships. She loved her children, each one having his or her own special connection with her. Of course, we perceived her work only as something that took her away from us. That made us remember our times with her like precious jewels of reminiscence.

Her love had no conditions or boundaries. Her laughter was like music and her sweet compassion was a blanket of comfort. She was a mother in every sense of the word and I found myself thinking that I would not do well in the world without her. As the years passed, I treasured her more. Eventually, my marriage began to fail, just when my mother was dying. My grief was beyond comprehension. I was given to believe that as a child, I was special. Now, I was going to lose the one person who knew and loved me best. I was afraid, uneducated, and not prepared to face survival.

She always told me, "you can do anything you want to do. You can be anything you want to be — nothing is impossible." It sounded plausible hearing her say that, but doing it was another matter.

Summoning every ounce of courage I had left, I enrolled in college to study nursing, not for altruistic reasons but for survival. My mother was very proud that I had chosen the same career she loved. She said it would come, the love of it. I couldn't love it because it was taking me away from being with her at a time when I needed to be with her most.

It was February and after months of dialysis and suffering, she completed her final journey to God, taking half of me with her. The day after her burial, I was separated from my husband. Two years later I graduated from nursing school. No longer able to cling to anything but myself, I was now faced with the real world: the working world, the 12-hour-shift world. I didn't think I could sustain the pressure and hard physical work.

I was working the night shift in labor and delivery, where physical demands were greater than I thought I could give. There were many mornings when I arrived home and just went to bed, clothes, shoes, and all. Something, I thought, was bound to give. I was tired and felt old. The stresses and physical demands are easier when you have youth on your side. I was an older beginner and felt the bumps like a jalopy without shock absorbers.

How I missed my mother. One night I was in the operating room alone. I had just scrubbed and donned my sterile gown, mask, and gloves. It was my duty that night to scrub on my first caesarean section. I prepared the operating room tables with instruments and medications. Sitting on a stool in this sterile environment, I waited alone for the patient to be brought in. The doctors usually arrived after the patient. Thoughts of my mother came to me. How I wished she could see me as a nurse, right here, right now. It was difficult but she was right. It had come to me, the love of it.

Almost praying, but in more of a conversational tone, I found myself asking her to show me a sign that she was happy in heaven, a sign that would be understood by me as being definitive.

The only sign I could think of was to ask her to close the hole in my heart. Then immediately, I took that request back, thinking it wrong to ask for something for myself. This isn't about you, I said to myself, this is about Mom. Saying I was sorry and didn't mean it, my request turned to anything of her choice.

You see, in my eyes, my mother was a saintly person. She had suffered in her life and bore her suffering with great dignity and grace. Surely, God would reward her with an eternity of happiness and peace. But, we never know and we always question, we who are of little faith. I felt she had a special connection to God and that He wouldn't refuse her a way to communicate with her daughter. Just as the patient was being wheeled in, I finished my "prayer" and ended it with, "just let me know that you're happy in heaven."

A month had passed and my prayer to my mother was completely forgotten. My mind-set was: no time, too busy, keep working. I was talking to a male nurse one day who worked with me in the unit. To my surprise, he told me that he also had a hole in his heart and like mine, it was never repaired. Well, I got out my stethoscope to show him how loud and swishy my murmur was. "I bet mine is louder than yours," I said. Putting the stethoscope over the area that would produce the loudest swish, I listened to my heart with disbelief. Tony was standing in front of me and the look on my face made him urgently question if I was alright. Tears started to flow down my face and I couldn't move the stethoscope away from my chest. For the first time in my life, I heard a normal heartbeat: thump thump, thump thump, thump thump. "It's gone! It's gone! You don't understand, it's gone!" I cried out. "You'd better go to the doctor," he said.

The next day I saw the Chief of Cardiology. He had been my cardiologist years ago when I had my children. A full extensive exam with echocardiogram and contrast was done. He then asked me into his office.

Sitting behind a big formal desk in a high-back chair, the doctor said, "I have been a cardiologist for 20 years, and I can tell you that I have never seen a ventricular septal defect close this late in life. If it closes it happens when you're a baby. This is so rare, it is reportable in a medical journal. I can't explain it." "I asked for it," I said. "My mother gave me that gift as a sign." Smiling, I said goodbye and left, knowing that Mom is happy in heaven.

The Vision Of Dad

Gina is a pretty, dark-haired nurse in her forties, who has experienced numerous unexplained occurrences. A woman of deep religious faith, she simply attributes her experience to gifts of Divine intervention. Here then, is one such story in her own words.

My father had planned on being a career soldier. But, he was injured in the Korean War, and became a paraplegic. Dad was always very patriotic, and loved all the fanfare surrounding the national holidays. Even as a kid, I remember all the decorations we'd put up around the house. He was very proud in spite of his injuries. As long as I can remember, he was in a wheelchair. He also suffered from bilateral trigeminal neuralgia, which made it difficult for him to smile. So for most of my life, I remember my father being sick and injured.

My father had surgery to remove a cancerous lung mass. My sister and I took turns going to Florida to care for him and my mother. My sister was there at the time when my husband received the call. Dad had died at home. I was devastated. I flew to Florida to be with my sister and to take care of the funeral arrangements.

My sister had brought Dad balloons for the July Fourth holiday. They were tied to a chair in the dining room. When I came into the dining room from the kitchen, the balloons began to move. My father was standing there tugging on the balloons. My father always used to wave with his fingers instead of with his hand. And there he was, standing there, tugging on the balloons with one hand and wiggling the fingers of his other hand. He was smiling. I said, "Oh my God." I ran to the kitchen and grabbed my sister and brought her in the room. She said, "How are you moving the balloons?" I said, "How can I be moving the balloons when I'm standing over here with you?" "What the heck?" she said. She didn't see him, but she saw the balloons being tugged. They weren't moving the way air moves them when you walk by. They were being tugged up and down. I saw him the whole time, the way I see you sitting here. He was standing erect and had a broad smile on his face. Softly, without looking at my sister, I said, "Daddy's there smiling at us and waving his fingers. He's moving the balloons."

Why some people can see these visions and others cannot, I can't explain. I recently had a patient who is in her 70's, and she told me about her sister, Rose. Millie had cared for her sister during a long illness. Rose had finally succumbed to the illness and died. A few nights afterward, Millie was awakened from a deep sleep. She said she had felt a presence. She looked towards the doorway and saw her sister standing in the doorway, looking beautiful and healthy. That was it, a momentary visit.

Other patients I have had demonstrated such behavior as looking up at the ceiling, pointing, laughing, and carrying on conversations with people I couldn't see. One patient, who was of Polish descent but had never spoken the language, was suddenly speaking fluent Polish to unseen visitors at her bedside. My patient was near death and her daughter was frustrated because her mother wouldn't speak English to her except on rare occasions. Her frustration lessened as she saw her mother draw closer to her "visitors" and appeared happier and more content.

These next two stories are about two people who saw heaven. You will undoubtedly be surprised that they sound like very similar experiences.

Are You Willing to Give This Up for Me?

I first met Gregg in 1993. It was a meeting I will never forget. I was working on the hospice team and one day a tall, handsome young man approached my desk. He introduced himself, saying, "Hi, I'm Gregg, one of the social workers. Got any cases for me?" I looked up and saw this young man smiling. He had such a positive attitude and his smile was the kind that tells you it's from the heart. We chatted some and the discussion soon led to a story about his accident. He sat down beside me and told me of his experience in which he saw what he believed to be heaven. "I don't know why I'm telling you this. I've never told anyone but my wife," he said.

Greg was the kind of social worker a hospice nurse dreams of having for his or her patients. He was one of the most dedicated and compassionate social workers I have ever worked with. But now I'm getting ahead of his story.

I recently contacted Gregg so that he could tell his story directly to you. He has the same dimpled smile, the same warm, compassionate style. And he wants you to hear his story. Here it is, in his own words:

> I had always been into bodybuilding. I was proud of the way I looked and because I was a competitive body-builder, I had to train every day. One day, while getting ready for an important competition, I was flexing in front of the mirror, doing all the different poses I'd be judged on. Suddenly, I heard a voice say, "Are you willing to give this up for me?" I ignored it because if I acknowledged hearing the voice, then I would have to acknowledge what it was asking me to do. I knew in my heart what was happening. And I also knew it wasn't my imagination. I continued posing, thinking it would go away. Again, I heard, "Are you willing to give this up for me?" The third time left me with no choice but to stop what I was doing. With a quiet resignation I just stood there looking into the mirror and said, "Thy will be done." I knew what the message meant: was I willing to give up my physical self, my love for my body, for the love of Him? I said yes.
>
> One week later, on July 21, 1989, I was in a car accident on I-95. My injuries were so extensive, they had to helicopter me to a trauma center. I had a broken foot, pelvis, and broken ribs. I tore my biceps, had torn my brain, and had a fractured skull and collapsed lungs. I

was in a coma for seven days. The doctor told my wife I had no better than a 50/50 chance of survival. "There's a good chance that he will be nonfunctioning for the rest of his life," the doctor said.

During the time when I was in a coma, I experienced being in a black void. If you can imagine being in outer space without stars, that is what it was like. It felt like I was floating or suspended. All of a sudden, I saw a white dot; it was that tiny. I was rushed to that white dot and all of a sudden, I was through it and out in this big wide field of grass and flowers. The grass was so green and it was so shimmering. It was greener than anything I've ever seen. The green that you see here on earth doesn't even come close. There isn't a green on this earth that is as beautiful as that. When I think about it, my heart...[shakes his head side to side]. And the flowers, nothing, nothing like it. And there were tulips of a whole bevy of different colors: purple, yellow, red, and white. They were all shimmering and translucent! All this time while I was in this field, there was a peace like you could never, ever imagine. And happiness — I mean I was happy as happy could be, and then [snap], in a split second I was there. I don't know how I got there but I was in front of this being. But the being was light, bright and white. The sun doesn't come close to the brightness of that light. It was pure, pure, pure. I looked and I was in awe. There was this being. I couldn't discern whether the being was male or female. It started communicating with me. It had a human form, but the light was so bright, they seemed to come together — the light was the being and vice versa. It's hard to describe. I felt as if I were the only person in the universe. It was that intense. It was like, you matter.

I was given a choice of whether I wanted to stay there or come back. At first, I was saying, my goodness, I want to stay here. But then thoughts of my wife and children came to me. Once I made the choice to come back, I was awake. From that point on, though, there was someone with me, who I'll call a sentry. He was always there with me like a powerful soldier. I couldn't see him, I could only feel him. And he was always at my left side. I felt very comfortable with the presence. The only thing I knew of that being, whatever it was, was that I knew I was loved, I was being cared for, and I was being watched. The only person that mattered was me. It was like a selfish presence. I was the only thing that mattered to it.

When I was being discharged six weeks later, this being that I called a sentry moved from the left side, where it always was, to the foot of my bed. I know it's here as we speak, but it's not as strong as the presence I felt in the hospital.

After the accident, there has been a constant molding. I was lying on the couch recuperating, and one day I was asked a question: "Do you know why you are here?" (It was just like the time before the accident. Only the question was different.) I said to myself, no. The voice said, "You are here to love. Everything flows from love."

God puts challenges in front of you. He wants you to be as perfect as possible. He wants you to come as close to Him as possible. This accident annihilated me physically, but spiritually, it made me robust. In effect, that's why we are here, to love and grow spiritually. I find myself loving people intensely now.

Whatever you're experiencing on this earth, I know you don't want to hear this, but there is no reason to hold on here. It's far better on the other side. You are actually home on the other side. The love that you experience down here is a joke compared to the love that is there. Our love is a shadow of what is there. You have to submit. Your journey through this short life is only to prepare you for the next life, which is total happiness and light.

Today, Gregg is a Eucharistic minister in the Catholic Church. He makes pastoral care visits to the sick and he travels to Staten Island to teach martial arts to children with disabilities. He faces each day with physical pain from nerve damage, but he always has a smile, and to meet him is to know that he is someone special.

This Has Not Transpired to Hurt, but to Heal

Grace is a warm, witty, and beautiful woman who also has a bit of the Irish whimsy in her. She is soulful, compassionate, serious, and funny at the same time. She has had three near-death experiences and all occurred while undergoing surgery.

It all started when she was kicked by a pony and developed osteomyelitis, a serious bone infection. With each surgery, they "lost" her for a short amount of time on the operating room table. I'll let Grace tell you the rest:

My first experience was an out-of-body experience where I was viewing myself on the operating table, watching everything and hearing their conversations. My grandmother, who had died when I was two years old, was with me. We were both viewing my physical body. She told me I had to wake up, saying, "It's not your time, I'm with you always." The next thing I remember is waking up in my hospital bed, and I could still perceive my grandmother. They thought I was this poor kid who was delusional and hallucinating, but I would know things through my grandmother. She'd say, "your Aunt Mary is coming and she's bringing you chocolates." A little while later, there was Aunt Mary with the chocolates.

With the second operation, I went through the tunnel and saw the light. The tunnel was permeable, not a solid structure. It felt as if there was energy there. The light itself was so pure, so warm. It was one love, like an energy I had never experienced before. In this light was the imagery of Christ. We spoke on a mental level. I could see my relatives in the background, what I call the welcoming committee. The imagery behind my relatives was in a field of nature: a brilliant waterfall, trees, brilliant flowers with colors I'd never seen before. It was very serene and tranquil.

Part of the communication I had with Christ was that this has not transpired to hurt, but to heal. I didn't want to come back. It was burdensome to come back. My soul had a choice at that point, but I realized that I still had a job to do, a responsibility that had to be fulfilled. It all happened with such split-second timing. It was so brilliant because I remember the feeling of understanding and comprehending that we're all connected, that we're all one and part of each other, that the true essence of existence is love and joy.

Having that veil of forgetfulness lifted for an instant left me with a total comprehension of what this life is supposed to be about. Everything does have a purpose and everything transpires for our soul's evolution. It was so peaceful, loving, compassionate: pure joy and ecstasy. It was a gift of absorption and knowledge.

My third near-death experience was again an out-of-body one. My grandmother was there again and said, "It's not your time. I'm always with you." This time, I saw her standing next to me in the recovery room when I woke up.

I know that in heaven, everything exists by creating what you want it to be. It's of your making. There was a movie made recently that depicted what heaven is like, Made in Heaven. It was like that.

People fear the process of dying and I think everyone forgets that we're here to be there. What they need to rejoice about is that they're going home. Where they are going is where they have always wanted to be. They're going down that Yellow Brick Road to Oz. The eternal love, joy, bliss, and fulfillment that is waiting for them is absolutely brilliant. That's what people have to be aware of. Both fear and pain can be transcended. What the soul is really yearning and longing for is to be united with God, the ultimate love.

Saint Peter is not up there with his book saying, "Oh it's in my book, you took a piece of gum when you were seven." Judgment is a self-examination in the presence of purity.

My one hopeful message to those of you reading this is: the best is yet to come. Think of the happiest, most joyful event or feeling you have ever experienced. Now multiply that a trillion times, and times that by eternity.

Gregg and Grace have told me their stories specifically as a message of hope for you. They truly believe that what they experienced was a vision of heaven in the presence of divine love. Heaven is there waiting for all of us who have faith and love enough to embrace it.

No matter what your religious beliefs are, there is always room for believing in something greater than yourself. Imagine that we can create our own heaven! Imagine being loved with such depth that it escapes human comprehension. Imagine being joined with loved ones in fields of flowers in a light that is brighter than the sun, and resting in pure joy and peace. How magnificent that moment of realization must be.

You are approaching the spring of your life, and like a dormant bud, your courage will rise to the occasion. You have all the resources within you to have the faith you need to embrace that which is your divine right—heaven. Like a bride who is being prepared before uniting with her soon-to-be husband, we too need to prepare for the union with God.

The last few weeks of life need special attention, the kind of attention that requires and deserves love, compassion, patience, and understanding. Now is the time to forgive and be forgiven. The soul desires peace in life as well as peace in physical death so that it may reside in peace for eternity.

Heaven is waiting, and you can go there when you are ready. You will know when the time is right for you. This preparation time is meant to give you comfort so you can care for your inner self, your spirituality. You matter. You are the only person in the universe right now, and it is my job to elevate your spirit within a clean, cared-for body, out of respect for Him, who has created you, and out of respect for the life you have courageously lived.

Chapter Eleven
Heaven Is Waiting

That which has grown from the earth to the earth,
But that which has sprung from heavenly seed, Back
to the heavenly realms returns.

Marcus Aurelius Antoninus

There are those who will have answered prayers, visions, and miracles. And there are many who are going on to the edge of heaven, as we all must sooner or later. For the many facing death in the near future, your prayers will also be answered in the form of courage, faith, and strength. Heaven is waiting. But heaven is also patient. Use this precious time to gather all the resources needed to help in your transition; this is a time for saying prayers, for meditation, and for having your spouse, children, and friends around you.

In this chapter, I will be showing your family how to give care that will preserve your privacy and self-respect, as well as help to reduce fear and anxiety. I will also be telling you what you need to know about what lies ahead. I need to give you, the reader, a name, because for me, this is the time when I draw closest to my patients. I need to "connect" with each person and each family. This may not be your real name or even your correct gender. But for now, you are my patient and whether you are Michael, Mary, Virginia, or George, I shall call you Kathryn. You are every man, woman, and child who has cancer and is dying.

This is your time, Kathryn; a holy time. Every effort shall be made to make sure you have everyone and everything you need to help make the transition. If you need a priest, minister, or rabbi, say so. If your grown children live out of state and you would like them here with you, say so. This is your time. Your request for them to come and be with you is as much for their sake as it is for yours. You don't want to leave them with the burden of regret. They need to be with you. They need to show you their respect and love. Let them come.

Use this time to reflect on your life and know that you have lived a life worth living. Your life is not over yet, and there is still time and love to share. And even when life is over for our bodies, death will be our new beginning. We want to bring you to that beginning as a whole person who has self-respect and dignity. Think of the Mountain of Visions and remember the stories of faith you have read. Draw closer to God as you are drawn closer to heaven, and have no fear because you are His own.

A way to make you feel that you are His own is through the care that is given to you. Giving care is an art. Giving care with meaning is a higher art. Everyone is capable of giving care with meaning, including your family. In fact, Kathryn, your family is probably the best choice in giving care because the love is already there. Meaningful care shows respect and consideration. It means paying attention to details like respecting your privacy, using a gentle touch, saying soft reassuring words, and creating a warm, gentle environment for you. The result of giving meaningful care is the preservation and elevation of your self respect and dignity. Meaningful care adds to your enjoyment of receiving care.

Let me give you an example: not all backrubs are alike. A backrub is given to relax you and also to make you feel loved. Would you feel loved if I came in, turned on the lights, and proceeded to give you a backrub with cold hands, cold lotion, and with the TV on? No, you wouldn't. And you wouldn't like the backrub, either. However, if I came in and said, "Kathryn, I'd like to give you a nice, warm backrub, let's turn off the TV, and I'll lower the lights," you'd be more receptive. I would warm my hands and use warmed scented lotion — your favorite. I would make sure the rest of your body is covered and kept warm. I would speak to you in a lowered, softer voice. I would take time. This is a backrub. This is giving care with meaning.

What about you, as the receiver of care? Can you accept your family doing this for you? Are you put off by being touched? These two issues are very important. If you cannot accept care without feeling guilty, then you will most likely not receive the care you need and deserve. There are feelings of guilt regarding being dependent on others and these feelings can lead to dismissal of care that might ultimately make you feel better. Getting past the guilt is a major accomplishment.

What about being touched? Let's talk about this for a moment. Touch can be a difficult issue because your cultural background and personal feelings may play a role in how you feel about this. Perhaps you have never allowed yourself to be seen undressed before. I do not underestimate the emotional and psychological impact of your concerns. And this can be a major issue if you are also uncomfortable or even frightened by the prospect of being touched. My answer to you is that care can and should be given in a very discreet manner. There is no need to be totally undressed at any time. While there are times when you will need a bath, this can be given in a gentle, private way that will preserve your dignity. And I believe that touch is very useful and necessary to communicate trust, love, and comfort. Once you get past the initial stage of discomfort, you will find yourself becoming more at ease with being touched in a healing, helping manner. Touch is important. Even allowing someone to hold your hand is very important. It connects you to the humanity of others in a way that communicates love and understanding.

Kathryn, having fear and anxiety is very natural and is expected. To combat fear, you need faith. To combat anxiety, you need meditation and perhaps medication. But I don't want you to become overpowered by these feelings. Now, if your anxiety is unmanageable, I think you should ask your doctor for antianxiety medication. I believe medication is necessary because it is unrealistic to expect that you will be able to handle this level of anxiety on your own. We will rate your anxiety the way we rated your pain level: on the 0 to 10 scale. If your anxiety is a level 5 or above, then we need to give you something like Xanax, Buspar, Ativan, or any of the other anxiolytic medications available. The medications will also help you sleep better at night.

Kathryn, I want to explain what usually occurs in general terms regarding the sequence of events leading up to death. Often, knowing what to expect can help in reducing at least some of your fear and anxiety. Then later, I will instruct your family on how to care for you, which will help them with their anxiety. Just remember, your family has been given the information they need so that they can help you.

Dying is a process that you feel — it doesn't just happen. When a person is dying, it is the result of a body system/organ failure. Usually a person senses what is happening. There is an increasing fatigue which develops and it is usually accompanied by a marked loss of appetite. The fatigue and lack of nutrition cause weakness, leading to an inability to walk or stand. The person then becomes bedbound due to the weakness. If nutrition decreases to only spoonfuls of custard or yogurt and fluid intake decreases to sips of fluids, then death will occur within a few days or weeks. Death is sometimes preceded by a coma.

If, however, a person is bedbound and is taking in enough nutrition and fluids, a reasonable level of conscious life can still be enjoyed and sustained in the company of one's family, provided pain and other symptoms are controlled.

There are important issues surrounding your care that you need to be aware of and that are directly related to your comfort and the way in which you want to die. What is most important is that you make your wishes known in your advance directives or in a living will. See (Chapter Five), if you have not already done so.

If you are depressed, we can give you an antidepressant. If you are very anxious, we can give you an antianxiety medication. Tell your family what you need and let them be your advocate to your doctor.

Nutrition is an important issue because there will probably be a time when you will experience difficulty in maintaining adequate nutrition and fluids to sustain your life. The lack of food and liquids will hasten your death. Palliative care, which is care to provide you comfort, does not preclude aggressive nutritional support, if this is what you want. An example of aggressive nutritional support is when you elect to have nutrition delivered via a tube (called enteral feeding) directly into your stomach or duodenum. This would be considered if you can no longer take food by mouth. These feedings consist of commercially prepared liquified food containing protein, carbohydrate, fat, vitamins, and minerals. Prolonging your life in this manner is your decision to make, and so that you can make an informed one, here are some considerations:

- If you want to have tube feedings (which can easily be done in the home), it will prevent further muscle wasting but it will not reverse your present condition. The feedings will provide you with a feeling of satiety and promote a sense of well-being and comfort.

- If you elect not to have tube feedings, muscle wasting will continue. You will also develop a dry mouth and dry tongue. Your mental awareness will decrease and your perception of pain will decrease. To keep you comfortable, we would use lubricants on your lips, and use a nonalcohol mouthwash. You would be given ice chips to suck on or a cold wet washcloth to suck on. Frequent mouth care would help the discomfort of a dry mouth and help with difficulties in swallowing.

There are different opinions among health professionals regarding nutritional support. Some feel that the aggressive tube feeding approach is equivalent to using "heroic" medical efforts, like placing a person on life support when he or she is unlikely to survive. Tube feedings will neither sustain life indefinitely nor prolong life substantially. I hardly consider tube feeding a "heroic" measure. When a patient can no longer swallow due to dehydration or tumor involvement, and he or she has a desire to feel satiated by the comfort of food, then we are just providing the patient with a normal life requirement. The only time that I wouldn't suggest starting tube feeding is if the patient is in immediate expectancy of death — within days. And, of course, it is always the wishes of the patient that take precedence over anyone else's suggestions.

So Kathryn, there are important decisions you need to make, and they should be in writing so your family and doctor can follow through with what you want or don't want done. What about a DNR order? This is a Do Not Resuscitate Order. You may have had one if you were hospitalized and told your doctor that is what you wanted. But did you know that a hospital DNR is different from a community DNR? In other words, a hospital DNR is not transferable to the home. Also, a DNR that is requested in your advance directives or in a living will is not sufficient to carry out your wishes. You will need a specific DNR document that can be obtained from your doctor, home care agency, hospice, or state health department.

If you were to die at home and you didn't have a community or nonhospital DNR document, the police and paramedics would initiate resuscitation, even five minutes after death had occurred. Resuscitation cannot be stopped, even if your family objects, and it would continue until they got you to the hospital. Only a hospital physician can determine the futility of the resuscitation and stop it.

If you do have a community DNR, which is at your request and signed by your doctor, your wishes would be carried out only if your family gives the document to the police when they arrive at your home. If your family can't find the document, the paramedics would begin cardiopulmonary resuscitation (CPR).

This is why it is very important to have your advance directives and DNR document, if that is what you choose, accessible to your family. Everyone should know where these papers are. In fact, they should be kept near you, perhaps in your night table or on your dresser.

Soon, I will be spending the rest of my time with your family. There are many things they need to know to help care for you. You are central in our minds and all of this is for your benefit. But before I go on to your family, there are still two issues we need to talk about.

First, earlier I said that if you need a priest, minister, rabbi, or other religious cleric you should say so. What if you were not religious in the past, should that prevent you from seeking help now? No. He or she is there to be called upon in your hours of need as well as in your hours of happiness. It is not uncommon for people to suddenly turn to God when they feel the end of their life is near. After all, it is He who is calling you. Never feel ashamed or embarrassed to ask your family to bring a representative of your faith to your side. This is when you need words of spiritual comfort so that you can begin to heal the assaults of life that have made their marks on you.

Second, I want you to look at your life, Kathryn. Are you so different from all the others in the world? Don't you think that everyone has made mistakes, made "wrong" decisions, or left a path they felt they were supposed to take? We're human. We are supposed to make mistakes. That's how we learn. Do you feel unfulfilled because you never accomplished what you thought you were meant to do? I could tell you at least five things I always thought I was meant to do because I thought I wanted to so much. Of course, they were at different times of my life. But, you know what? Nursing and becoming an author weren't among them. My dreams were entirely unrelated to what I'm doing now.

You became who you are because that is who you were supposed to be. Whether you are a housewife or a career woman, you are what was intended. Our purpose isn't to be something; it is to be somebody. And you are somebody. You have influenced people all your life, and mostly you are unaware of your impact. You may have children. Your children will carry on your teachings, which will be handed down perhaps for generations. You have planted your seed. You have seen and lived life. And of all the people in the world, there is not one who is greater than another. It is not position that makes for success, but disposition.

You can go in peace, Kathryn. There is nothing that should lead you to believe that you have not succeeded in your life. It takes courage to live and courage to die. You have shown what you're made of. You have made a difference in this world, and that difference will continue on.

Family Members Gather Around: Let's Talk

I, too, have lost loved ones. I know what you are going through. You need care and understanding as much as Kathryn does. That is why all of you need to help each other through this difficult time. Make sure you get enough rest. Make sure you eat well. Support one another as much as you can. You have a tremendous gift to give - the gift of loving care.

You are stronger than you could imagine. That strength is what is going to help you now. Trust in your beliefs and try not to become despondent over "little failures." The expectation of perfection leads to unwarranted stress. Do the best you can. Show Kathryn as much love as you can. That will be more than enough. You are not alone. There are hundreds of thousands of families presently in the same situation. And, remember, there are home care, hospice, community, and American Cancer Society resources to help you. You will nonetheless be stressed because changes are coming and you will need each other's love, support, and understanding. You have to keep your wits about you. You're going to be tired, irritable, and short-tempered. Try to keep calm. You will know ahead of time what to expect and what you can do. It is most important that you keep organized. Find a routine. Routines limit stress.

Now is the time to consider getting help in the home. Home care is good, but remember that home care is under managed care, so if Kathryn suddenly takes a turn for the worse, you may find yourselves fighting for nursing visits and home health aide visits. You can always start out with home care, then switch to hospice care. Once you choose hospice, and this can be done six months before an anticipated death, managed care is no longer involved. Hospice would take over the care management completely. If at any time you feel you can't manage Kathryn's care on your own, then please do not hesitate to call your local hospice. There will be a lot of questions you will have along the way, and they can help answer them. Hopefully, I will be able to answer most of your questions by telling you about the primary aspects of care.

Reconciliations

You need to have everything in place so that Kathryn's transition can occur in a comforting and loving environment. This is often easier said than done. Not every family has supportive members. There may be long-standing divisions between you. For your sake and Kathryn's, this would be a good time for reconciliation. If there is a division between close relatives, it could have an impact on whether or not Kathryn wishes to remain at home and how Kathryn views herself during her dying stage. She may feel she has failed in her life. She may feel responsible. If words were never spoken after a division, it doesn't mean it was forgotten. Life is too short and no event is more important than leaving this world in peace. Whatever it takes, try to make it happen. Let me tell you a story.

My father had been ill for a long time, for years. He had children by another marriage, which was unknown to me until I was an adult. I know he must have thought about them, but he never spoke of them and had not seen them for thirty years.

I was very young when my "cousin" came to live with us for a year. He was about 10 years my senior. That was a wonderful year for me, and I became very attached to Richard. He was like a brother to me. He was a brother. And for many years after he left our home, I wondered what had happened to him. He had just disappeared into military service. Our time together was short, but it made a lasting impression on me. It made such an impression that when I was told he was my brother, I knew I had to find him for my father's sake. I was married then and had my own responsibilities and obligations, but I knew I had to do this for Dad. I sensed that he did not have much time left.

A friend's husband was a detective, so I asked for help — just an address and phone number. Within 24 hours, the information was in my hands. I made the call. I drove out of state to see him. While driving down a street in that strange town, I spotted a man walking towards the car. He looked just like my dad, only younger. I stopped the car, threw open the door, and he and I were running towards each other at the same time. What a day that was!

I made a call to our father and told him what I had done. In a slow, deliberate voice, he said, "I could kill you for this." Not wanting Richard to know what was said, I calmly replied, "OK Dad," and hung up. I invited Richard to spend a weekend with me at my home, and he accepted. I called Dad and asked if he wanted to see Richard. "Alright, bring him over," he said. Both my parents were initially very upset. I didn't mean to interfere, but I thought it would help Dad if he saw Richard even once.

The reunion wasn't what I expected. Richard put his arms around his father and, in effect, forgave him. Dad couldn't take his eyes off his son. It wasn't tense or harrowing. It was peaceful and loving. Dad said later that he was glad he came. He didn't have to tell me. I saw it on his face. Dad died a few months later. During the wake and funeral, my brother, Richard, didn't leave my side. Six years later, Richard also died, of colon cancer.

The thought of opening family closets is abhorrent because of the uncertainty of what will happen. Sure, I was scared. My family did not support me in the beginning. I was yelled at and thought of as a fool. But, in my heart I knew I was doing the right thing. Maybe it's not right for every family. I can't really answer that. The fact is, it's worth the risk.

I told you this story because it is relevant for you and your family. Believe me, I understand family divisions. And when I say "do whatever you can," I really mean it. Reconciliation heals old wounds. Old wounds shouldn't go to the grave.

Getting Ready

The family's emotions are understandably high at this time. All of you will need to keep organized and make sure you are getting enough sleep. Rotate your time with Kathryn, if you can. One person doing all the care during the day is a hardship because there will be nights that Kathryn will require attention as well.

Sometime around the initial stage of dying (which I will deal with later) is when you should consider getting hospice involved. Hospice will provide everything you need to care for Kathryn, including pain medication, oxygen, a hospital bed, a physician, expert nursing care, and a home health aide for personal care. Anything you need is covered under your hospice benefits within your medical plan. I strongly encourage you to call hospice. They can give you the emotional and physical support you urgently need.

You will begin to see changes in Kathryn's physical condition as well as in her mental condition. These are end-of-life changes.

End-of-life changes occur in sequential stages. A person could be bedbound for months as a consequence of multiple factors like paralysis, cardiac disease, or renal failure coupled with end stage cancer disease. There are other instances where a person remains ambulatory but, because of a rapid decline, becomes bedbound for a week or several weeks prior to dying. In other words, the decline can occur slowly or rapidly, depending on many factors such as the advancing state of the disease and the person's physical, emotional, and psychological condition. The will to live also affects the rate of decline since it is a significant factor in prolonging life.

Since changes can occur unexpectedly, the family needs to be ready to cope with the many decisions and demands concerning Kathryn's care. You need to know what to do and when to do it. I'll discuss the care with you in the stages that coincide with what I have determined to be the stages of dying. There are no steadfast rules to follow. This is meant to be a general guide to help you go through it together. I know you can do this. Try to remain strong and keep your courage. Remember to divide care responsibilities so as not to overburden a single family member. Also, see that each caregiver gets a day or two off to pursue his or her own recreation/activities.   Most importantly, be sure everyone receives a proper amount of rest. Hospice can fill in the gaps for you.

The Initial Stage

I call this the initial stage because there will be noticeable signs and symptoms that will necessitate making changes in your environment, i.e. getting equipment and supplies, gathering family around, and providing religious support, if needed. This initial stage is perceptible. It occurs as a marked change in a person's condition. It usually occurs suddenly and is quickly followed by a rapid physical decline, which then stops at a plateau level. The initial stage is the first stage of dying and it can last for weeks, or months.

Signs and Symptoms

Kathryn will have difficulty keeping her balance when walking, or will lose her balance when getting up from a chair. You will notice a progressive decrease in her weight. She'll complain that she has no appetite. She'll start to refuse to eat food on most occasions. She'll complain of excessive fatigue. You will notice her sleeping a lot during the day. There may be increased pain, nausea, dry heaves or vomiting, all of which can be mitigated with the proper medications. (Refer to Chapters Three and Seven.) Constipation is often a problem at this time because of dehydration, decreased food and fluids, and drug side-effects.   Also, Kathryn will start to look differently to you.   She'll look pale, drawn, lethargic, depressed, and possibly anxious. You will probably see increased irritability.

A Time to Change the Environment

The first thing you need to consider is Kathryn's room. What kind of bed is she sleeping in? Is the bathroom close by? Are these rooms "safe" given her particular condition. Safety refers to objects or furniture in the path where she may walk. She might be prone to falls, so you want to keep pathways clear with no scatter rugs to trip on.

The Room

As always, her room should be bright and cheery. A room with shades drawn during the day will foster a deepening depression and feelings of increased isolation. Get out grandma's comforters or any favorite blankets that Kathryn likes. If you can, set up a TV, radio, VCR and/or a CD player so she can enjoy movies and music. Put family pictures around so she can see them. Install a telephone on her night table where she can reach it so she can receive and make calls. Most people who are very ill are afraid of the dark and fear going to sleep at night. Put night lights in all of the bedroom electrical sockets.

The room location is an important consideration for all of you. If her bedroom is upstairs, but the kitchen is downstairs, there could be problems. She's going to need a lot of attention, both physical and emotional. If her room is upstairs, you, the caregiver, are going to have to climb those stairs many times a day with medications, fluids, foods, and to give her a bath, and to help her to the toilet, etc. Also, Kathryn will feel isolated from the rest of the family. This is what we want to avoid. So, if at all possible, move her to a room in close proximity to the mainstream of life in the house, where she can hear conversations and be part of them. Convert a den or dining room to a temporary bedroom. If she needs privacy, put up a screen. Her quality of life depends on being with you, not by herself. Her surroundings should be quiet enough for her to rest when she wants to, but not isolating.

The Bed

If Kathryn can walk with assistance, you don't need a hospital bed. Someone should be able to accompany her to the bathroom and then take her back to bed. If, however, she is too weak to walk to the bathroom even with assistance, then you should rent an electric hospital bed with an air mattress, side rails, and a trapeze so she can change positions without assistance. This is very important for several reasons. Kathryn needs as much autonomy and comfort as she can get. An electric hospital bed has remote controls, which she can use to change her position without asking for help.

The hospital bed's side rails do not need to be up unless Kathryn is exhibiting confusion. Sometimes when a narcotic is given for pain there will be some confusion, especially at night. For this reason, to avoid the possibility of falls, it is preferable to use the side rails when confusion is exhibited.

The air mattress or egg crate mattress on a hospital bed is there to prevent Kathryn's skin from breaking down. Bedsores can develop quickly from the pressure of the body lying in one position too long. Kathryn will be prone to infection due to a decrease in her immune system's ability to fight. A small break in the skin often leads to bedsores. Remember to give Kathryn a way of getting your attention if she should need you. A bell or a portable intercom, the same that is used for a baby's room, would do well.

A hospital bed for the patient is important for the caregivers as well. A caregiver can easily injure his or her back if it is necessary to turn, pull, or lift Kathryn in a regular bed that requires bending while performing these tasks.

Some people resist the hospital bed because it has negative connotations. The bed signals a greater severity of illness and some view it as threatening. But the benefits of having a hospital bed can be substantial to both the patient and the caregivers. It can increase the safety, autonomy, independence, and comfort of the patient. For the caregivers, it means being able to give care with reduced risk of injury, and less involvement in doing tasks that the patient can now do by himself or herself.

Who Will Pay for the Bed?

Most insurances have coverage for rentals of durable medical equipment, which includes the bed, overhead trapeze, side rails, wheelchairs, and bedside commodes. The American Cancer Society can pay for the equipment or if you have hospice, they will provide these things for you.

Kathryn's Physical Care

Kathryn's physical care will depend on her physical condition. Because the initial stage is a period of significant decline, you will have to adjust the care needs as the decline progresses. Remember, her doctor should be informed when there is a change like pain, not eating, constipation, severe swelling in the legs, nausea, vomiting or difficulty breathing, confusion, and fever. It is always best to notify the doctor of any changes in her condition.

Also remember, you do not have to go through this alone. Call hospice care. They provide the nurse, aide, pastoral care (spiritual care), Intravenous teams, as well as a staff physician.

Bathing

As long as Kathryn can stand without assistance and walk without help, she can take a shower, but someone should be with her in the bathroom. A rubber bath mat should be placed in the bathtub to prevent slipping. If she cannot walk on her own, she will need to be bathed in bed.

At first, she may resist your attempts to help because she may be angry, feel she is a burden, or be depressed. Continue your efforts to give her a bath/shower because if she is kept clean, she will feel healthier and have an increased feeling of well-being. Feeling clean may even help her to eat and drink. Remember, cleanliness affects attitude, outlook, and self-esteem. When she is no longer able to stand or walk without assistance, the bed bath becomes the method of choice for cleanliness.

The Bed Bath

This is easy to do. First, gather your supplies: a large basin, two towels, soap, a washcloth, and a small bedside table or stand. Make the water hot, but not hot enough to burn. Remove her clothing, but cover her completely with a sheet or blanket. Let her do as much by herself as possible. If she can't help, then you'll have to do it all. Start from the head down. Never keep her uncovered. When you wash an arm, place one towel under her arm, keeping the rest of her body covered. Just wash and dry one body part at a time and then cover her. When you wash her back, place the hot washcloth against her skin and leave it there awhile. The heat is soothing. Private parts of the body are washed last with new water. After the bath, use lotion on her feet, hands, elbows, and back. She probably will be dehydrated and you want her skin soft to prevent cracking. Face and hands should be washed at least two times a day.

Washing the Hair

This is as important as giving a bath. There is an easy way to do this if she can't get out of bed. Lie her across the bed with her head elevated by pillows. Take a trash bag and, without opening it, lay it under her head and shoulders so it drapes down over the side of the bed into a bucket on the floor. You'll need a large water pitcher and shampoo. Her head should be a little off the pillows to prevent the water from running towards her back. That's it. It works very well. Towel dry and use a blow dryer so her hair isn't wet. She will feel so much better now that she's bathed and has had her hair washed. And you'll feel better at having given her the gift of feeling clean and happy. Also, use this as a time for conversation and an exchange of love!

If she is too ill to have her hair washed this way, try using a washcloth with shampoo and a little water. Take off the excess shampoo with a moistened washcloth and dry with a towel.

Bedsores

The bath presents an opportunity to check her skin. This is very important because we want to make sure she doesn't develop bedsores. Check her elbows, back, coccyx (tail bone) area, hips, and the heels of her feet. These areas break down first. An ulcer can develop into a serious infection and sepsis. Look for reddened areas. A prolonged reddened area means a stage I ulcer (bedsore). If you see this redness, pad or protect the affected areas with pillows. She will need to be turned every 2 to 4 hours to alleviate the pressure from these areas. The egg crate mattress or an air mattress helps. Be sure to call the doctor to notify. He may want to order a cream medication.

Mouth Care

This is given in the morning and evening. If she has a dry mouth, use nonalcohol rinses frequently to help refresh her. If she can't brush her own teeth, use a washcloth dipped in a mouth- wash and gently clean her teeth and gently wipe the inside of the mouth.

Nails

Keep her nails short so she doesn't scratch herself or get dirt under them. The toenails should be short also. Do not cut her nails yourself if Kathryn is a diabetic. There are podiatrists who make house calls. This is covered under Medicare. Also check with your other insurance carrier.

Nutrition

Getting nutrition is often a problem, especially when Kathryn starts refusing to eat most meals. If she is nauseous, ask the doctor for an antinausea medication like the ones described in Chapter Three. If the complaint is that she has no appetite, then ask the doctor for an appetite stimulant like Megace or Periactin.

If Kathryn can't eat solid food, call the doctor. The doctor may put her on a liquid drink like Ensure or Boost or any other commercial formula. Also consider talking to Kathryn and the doctor about tube feedings. Tube feedings are usually a last resort. Otherwise try small frequent feedings, 4 to 6 times a day. Yogurt, custards, soups, cold fruit cut in pieces, anything she will eat. Try to always feed her favorite foods — things she loves to eat. There are usually no dietary restrictions since she isn't taking in enough quantity to be harmful. Check with the doctor whenever you try anything new and especially if she is a diabetic.

The issue of nutrition often becomes a battleground of wills. Culture plays a large role in this. If your cultural and ethnic background dictates that large hearty meals have a high priority in family life, then you will most likely become very anxious when Kathryn can no longer eat as she used to. Your natural desire to "push" food is now met with Kathryn's resistance. This can cause tension, anxiety, and frustration for everyone in the family.

The acceptance of Kathryn as she is now, no longer wanting to eat, (after all else has failed), is the acceptance of the fact that she is dying. This acceptance will be very difficult for you. Try to understand that she is not being difficult. She just can't eat. Her body is sending signals that it is time to start shutting down. No stimulant, pleading, or begging can reverse this. The main objective now is to keep her as comfortable as possible. If she refuses nutrition, you shouldn't force her to take it.

Fluids

Fluids are in the same category as food. Often, Kathryn will not be able to drink enough fluids to sustain adequate hydration. If she is only taking sips of fluids, this will not be enough for her. Her mucous membranes will dry up, giving her a very dry mouth and cracked lips, and her level of consciousness will eventually decrease into a somewhat semiconscious state. Mouth care during this period is very important in keeping her comfortable. Offer her ice chips and use petroleum-based lip balm on her lips.

There are different opinions regarding artificial hydration — the use of intravenous fluids — when a person can no longer drink. I have advocated hydration in the home for my patients who were alert and oriented. Fluids can help sustain that level of consciousness and increase overall comfort.

There are other professionals who feel that dehydration will decrease the pain sensation and induce mental clouding. I agree that mental clouding results from dehydration. But I do not agree that it decreases the pain sensation. A person under deep anesthesia still feels pain. That is how the anesthesiologist controls the levels of anesthesia, by monitoring the signs of pain: increased respiration, increased heart rate, increased blood pressure, etc. A person may look pain-free, but if he or she is unable to communicate, we shouldn't assume that he or she isn't having pain. That is why we still give pain medication around the clock whether a patient is sleeping or not.

Artificial hydration can be accomplished easily by either using a small catheter that is inserted into a vein or by inserting a smaller catheter under the skin. Hydration could be regulated to give just enough fluids for comfort, i.e. to keep the mucous membranes from drying. Most certified home health agencies have an infusion department with special Intravenous teams that come to the home for this and other purposes.

Bowels

Kathryn's bowel habits will change. As she takes in less food, there will be fewer bowel movements. Constipation becomes a problem because the rhythmic motion of the bowel slows down and there is less fluid in the bowel to promote evacuation. A bowel obstruction can occur, causing nausea, vomiting, and abdominal rigidity. Call the doctor and ask for a bowel regimen — stool softeners or a mild laxative if no bowel movement occurs in 2 to 3 days. Sometimes an impaction can occur which requires manual removal of feces. The doctor can advise on what to do. Sometimes a fleet or oil enema is all that is needed.

Bladder

If Kathryn is taking in less fluids, she will have less urinary output. If, however, she is able to drink or if she is getting intravenous fluids, she should be putting out normal amounts of urine. Her urine output should be measured if she can urinate in a bedpan or commode. She should be putting out at least 30 cc's an hour. Sometimes a Foley catheter is inserted when a patient is bedbound. Its purpose is to monitor urinary output and to protect the patient from lying in a urine-soaked bed if he or she should lose bladder control. A Foley catheter is not absolutely necessary unless there is little output and she is drinking or on IV fluids.

Low fluid output combined with normal fluid input would mean that her bladder is full and we would have to release the urine. If she has less than 30 cc's an hour of output, she could be exhibiting signs of renal shutdown, or failure. If there is little or no urinary output, then her death could occur within days, a stage which would be characterized by a decrease in mental awareness and then a coma.

Giving Medications

This can be a confusing task, especially if there are different medications for different times of the day. It is very useful to get a mediplanner from the drugstore. This is a plastic container which holds medications for an entire week; each day is divided into morning, noon, evening, and bedtime. The mediplanner will save you time, keep you organized, ensure that the proper medications are given, and help decrease your anxiety.

Some medications can be crushed or converted to a liquid form. But never crush the extended-release form of morphine. This will result in overdosing. Check with your doctor if Kathryn experiences difficulty in swallowing medications. Do not administer crushed medication without the consent of her doctor.

Keep the pain scale rating flow sheet posted by Kathryn's bed. (See Appendix 7 for sample) You should know what to do now from Chapters Six and Seven. Just monitor her pain levels and if she goes to a level 5, call the doctor. If she cannot swallow her pain medication, consult her doctor, who may tell you to give it rectally with a little mineral oil or butter on the pill.

Keep a medication chart to write down which medications she is receiving and at which time of day they are to be given. One person should be responsible for giving medications. Keep the chart with the mediplanner.

Make sure you have enough medication on hand and reorder before you run out. Nothing is more distressing than running out of morphine at midnight when the patient is in pain.

The same is true for any supplies you may need. If she has a colostomy, you will want to order enough flanges and bags in case of emergencies. Save the boxes because the reorder numbers are on them. Most pharmacies do not carry ostomy supplies. You'll need to order directly from a manufacturer like Hollister or from a surgical supply company. It can take 2 to 3 days for delivery at times, so be prepared. Most hospitals have an ostomy nurse specialist on staff. Use that resource to help you with any questions concerning ostomy care. If you have hospice, they would supply the needed supplies.

Intravenous Pain Management

The time to consider an intravenous drip for pain management is when Kathryn has difficulty swallowing and when the pain is increasing faster than it can be controlled with pills. An intravenous drip of morphine or Dilaudid is very effective. It can be supplemented by allowing Kathryn to access a control switch called a bolus button to deliver a preset amount of extra medication, should she have breakthrough pain. The Intravenous team would monitor how many times she requested a bolus. Only a given amount of boluses are programmed to deliver medication within a given time period. If she is trying to bolus for more medication than is programmed to release within that given time period, it would show in the equipment. The doctor would then be called by the Intravenous team to increase the standing dose.

The Plateau Stage

The initial stage of decline often plateaus and there is a period of relative stability — the plateau stage. This plateau stage is usually short in duration, lasting from a few days to a few weeks. The plateau stage then rapidly declines into the imminent stage, lasting from hours to days.

The Imminent Stage

Signs and symptoms of the imminent stage are varied, and may include all or some of these following symptoms. Kathryn will begin to show increased *confusion*. She may not recognize familiar faces. She may not understand what is being said to her. She will *lose bowel and bladder control*. She will be *restless, agitated, and incoherent*. You will notice that her fingertips and toes are *turning a bluish color*, which may extend to the palms, fingers, and the soles of her feet. There is usually an *increased difficulty in breathing*. There may be some *bleeding* from any orifice in her body. Sometimes the bleeding can be heavy, but this is not common. Bleeding occurs in some instances when the person has had extensive chemotherapy and the platelet count decreases to a level in which the blood is no longer clotting. With all the patients I have had, there were only two people who had bleeding. If bleeding does occur, use dark colored towels to clean the area. The sight of blood can be frightening to anyone. Dark colored towels make the blood less visible.

What You Can Do for Her

- Call her doctor, ask for suggestions, explain her condition/symptoms.

- You must constantly reassure her that she is not alone. She will still have the capacity to hear you. Talk to her. Touch and stroke her. If she experiences confusion, orient her to reality. Tell her where she is and who is with her.

- Keep her body clean and free from urine and feces. Get Chux pads from the pharmacy and keep clean ones under her.

- To calm her restlessness and agitation, you can try reading or talking to her about the happy memories she has given you. If patients of mine liked angels, I would read angel stories to them. It had a calming effect on both of us.

- If Kathryn says she sees people coming or tells you she hears music, listen to her. It has been my experience that dying people are privileged to see visions that cannot be experienced by those of us who are to remain behind. Remember, she is crossing over now and she is being transferred from your hands to the hands of those who have gone before her. Typically, these visions are comforting to the dying, usually taking the form of a close, deceased relative. Not everyone experiences this, but it usually occurs within a week of dying. I believe these visions to be real.

- If she is experiencing difficulty in breathing, call the doctor. He can order oxygen to be brought into the home. Most insurances require a blood gas test or pulse oximter to measure oxyhemoglobin in the blood before oxygen is given. A blood gas test cannot be done in the home, but oximetry can, and it only takes 30 seconds for a reading.

- Difficulty in breathing can progress into what is called agonal breathing. The mouth opens wide in attempts to get air. Sometimes a little morphine helps to relieve the anxiety associated with inability to get enough air. Even with oxygen being administered, there can be difficulty in breathing.

- Sometimes, having a small fan running (about three feet away) from the top of a dresser can make her feel better because she can feel the air being moved around. She will need to be monitored for chills or feeling cold. If she's sweating, she's too hot. If her skin feels cool, she may be cold, so cover her with another blanket.

- If there is an increase in fluid collection in the lungs, you will hear gurgling. This too can be helped. Call the doctor, who can give a prescription for Atropine. Atropine 0.4 mg can be given subcutaneously (under the skin) by injection. The atropine helps in suppressing the production of saliva and secretions from the throat and lungs.

- If there is any bleeding, use dark brown or black towels to clean her. It can be frightening to see blood. She can't see it when you use dark towels.

The Final Point of Crossing Over

Here we are, at the final point of crossing over from this world to the next. I have been with you for about two years now. Every thought and every feeling has passed through me like changing seasons. There were days when I have cried writing about patients I have had. There were days I have cried for you, knowing what you're going through. I have prayed every day before beginning to write, asking for help to bring you the information you need in a way that would convey my true concern and compassion. Through this, I have grown closer to my family for their sacrifices, closer to God for giving me hope, and closer to you because you were with me for so long. I have done the very best I could do. I hope you feel that your journey with me was helpful.

I believe there are purposes in life. Everyone has one. Success isn't measured by money or position. Success is measured by what we give to others, what we learn, and what changes we make to improve ourselves and those around us. We are all struggling through life together. Make your life count. Make your death count. It all matters.

Heaven is waiting and we need to help Kathryn through this last stage. This last vigil can be a profound experience for all of you. Don't be afraid to handle her, talk to her, or say prayers for her. It's what she needs. This is all part of comfort care. If she has children, let them come in to be with her. They, too, need to say good-bye. Tell her it's alright to leave. Let her know that you will be alright. She may look unresponsive, but she can hear you. She can still perceive your voice and touch, so talk to her and hold her hand. You can tell her you love her dearly and that she was a good wife and mother, that you will never forget her and that only good things await her. Tell her not to be afraid. You have given Kathryn the greatest gift of all - dying at home, family care, love and support. You will have no regrets.

Afterward

The grief of losing a loved one will be with you a long time. You may feel frightened and alone. There may be anger. You may cry for no apparent reason. You may feel depressed and lethargic. These are all normal responses to grief. Take one day at a time, one thought at a time. Eventually, your grief will be transformed into strength. You will be able to think of your loved one with happiness instead of tears. You will go on because that is what we all have to do. You still have things to learn and accomplish. Your mission may still be in front of you. So hold on and trust that you will be helped when you need it. Seek out your support. You have a tremendous capacity for courage and strength right inside your own being and, in my view, your loved one will always be right there beside you.

You will now carry with you not only his or her memory, but you will have the firm conviction that you have done everything possible to make your lives richly fulfilling for all concerned. And this achievement, my dear friends, will be with you all the days of your life. Caring for a loved one is a very noble deed. You will have no regrets. When it is time for you to die, I pray it will be the same for you, just as I pray it will be that way for me.

We are all connected. The meaning of life is you, what you make of it and what you bring to it. It is that simple and that complex. You matter, just like Kathryn matters and George or John. We all carry within us the meaning of life.

As I have sat here, looking out my second story window, I could see directly into the tops of the trees. I have watched the birds come and go, seen dark clouds and clear skies, sunny days and rainy days. I have changed with the changing seasons. A picture of my mother sits in front of me, her smile reminiscent of her love and courage. She has given me the strength to do this work every day. They are still with us, the ones we've loved who have crossed over. And life will go on after we, too, are gone. Hopefully our journey together has given you renewed faith, a stronger love of philosophy, a greater love for your family, and a firm conviction that we all will be going home to a heightened glory too sublime to comprehend. Good-bye, and know that I am with you every step of the way. One breath from Him upon our lips is all we ask.

One Breath from Him upon Your Lips

You don't know me, but I have watched you.
I have walked your journey many times before.
You don't know me, yet I was there.

Icy winters and raging winds blew across my face
As I looked to heaven and earthly domains
In search of your relief.

Your frail, sick and frightened being
Changed before my very eyes -
One breath from Him upon your lips.

I was there and saw it happen;
The hope of mankind in your eyes,
An outstretched hand to Heaven's light.

It wasn't me you saw this day
But secret visions of things to come;
Secrets you could not impart.

One breath from Him upon your lips
Set forth four winds to lift your soul
In heightened glory too sublime.

One breath from Him upon your lips -
I knew then, you were free.

Love Nancy

Appendix Chapter 1

American Cancer Society
1599 Clinton Road, NE
Atlanta, GA 30329
(800)ACS-2345
Provides counseling, education, and information.
Reimbursement towards travel, medical supplies, and
financial assistance in some areas.

American Society of Clinical Oncology
225 Reinakers Lane, Suite 650
Alexandria, VA 22314
(703)299-0150
Has information by leading cancer professionals on
cancer and clinical trials.

Cancer Care
1180 Avenue of the Americas
New York, NY 10036
(212)221-3300
Counseling, financial assistance in some areas, telecon-
ferencing with health experts, educational resources.

Cancer Research Institute
681 Fifth Avenue
New York, NY 10022
(800)99-CANCER
Information on clinical trials. Funds research at univer-
sities and laboratories. Provides a 50-page health book:
What to do if Cancer Strikes, $2.00 S/H charge.

Candlelighters Childhood Cancer Foundation
7910 Woodmont Avenue, Suite 460
Bethesda, MD 20814
(800)366-2223
Peer support, counseling, information on pain
management.

National Family Caregivers Association
9621 East Bexhell Drive
Kensington, MD 20895-3104
(800)896-3650
Provides counseling, support groups, education, and information.

Appendix Chapter 2

For publications from Health Care Financing Administration call: (410)786-3183

- *Medicare Risk Plans and the Point of Service Benefit Questions and Answers.*

- *1999-2000 Medicare Handbook.*

- *Medicare Beneficiary Advisory Bulletin: (HMO) Know Your Rights 10934.*

*   *   *   *   *

- Medicare Hotline 1-800-638-6833.

- For information on the Hill-Burton Uncompensated Division of Facilities Compliance and Recovery HRSA, HHS, contact Suite 520, Twinbrook Metro Plaza, 12300 Twinbrook Parkway, Rockville, Maryland 20852 (301)443-5656 or 1-800-638-0472 or 1-800-492-0359 (for callers outside of Maryland).

- Supplemental Security Income — SSI is a program for financial aid to persons 65 or older and for the blind or disabled who are in need of financial assistance. 1-800-772-1213.

- Eldercare Locator has information about services avaiable to older persons living within the U.S. 1-800-677-1116.

- AARP
601 E. Street, NW,
Washington, D.C. 20049
(202)434-2277.

- Online Resource
  WWW.Medicare.gov
  Medicare Health Plans. Important contacts.
  Publications. Wellness. Nursing Homes.
  Medicare questions and answers.
  Medicare beneficiary outreach calendar.

Appendix Chapter 5

1995 National Homecare and Hospice Directory —

- 815-page national guide to homecare and hospice agencies. Your local library or medical book store should have this. If not, contact the National Association for Homecare, 519 C Street, NE, Washington, DC 20002-5809 - (202)547-7424.

- *AARP Pharmacy Service Ostomy and Incontinence* Catalog. Free — call 1-800-284-4788 Dept. 617706.

- Dignity® Plus — products for secure dry comfort. For information on bladder care management 1-800-631-5270.

- Lifeline® — 1-800-543-3546. A hands-free telephone emergency response system. (Important for someone living alone.)

- Cancer Care Teleconferences — this is a way for you to get the latest information on treatment from leading experts. Teleconferences are free. Prior registration is required. For more information call Cancer Care Counseling line at 1-800-813HOPE or call their national office at (212)302-2400.

- *Managing Your Colostomy* — 12-page booklet from Hollister. Along with the booklet, an educational video is available. For a free copy, call 1-800-323-4060 (U.S.), 1-800-263-7400 (Canada), (708)680-1000 (international)

- Additional educational materials and videos on home health care are available from:
  Hollister Incorporated
  2000 Hollister Drive
  Libertyville, Illinois 60048

Booklets for Cancer Patients/Families from the National Cancer Institute

The following information is free of charge. Call 1-800-4Cancer or write to:

Office of Cancer Communications
National Cancer Institute
Building 31, Room 10A24
Bethesda, MD 20892

- Advanced Cancer: Living Each Day

- Eating Hints: Recipes and Tips for Better Nutrition During Cancer Treatment

- Radiation Therapy and You: A Guide to Self-Help During Treatment

- What Are Clinical Trials All About?

- When Cancer Recurs: Meeting the Challenge Again

- Answers to Your Questions About Metastatic Cancer

Other Booklets Available from the National Cancer Institute:

What you need to know about:	Publication number
Lung Cancer	93-1553
Brain Tumors	93-1558
Cancer of the Bone	93-1571
Cancer of the Cervix	91-2047
Kidney Cancer	91-1569

Bladder Cancer	93-1559
Melanoma	93-1563
Non-Hodgkins Lymphomas	93-1567
Cancer of the Uterus	93-1562
Mastectomy — A Treatment for Breast Cancer	91-658

American Cancer Society — 1-800-ACS 2345.
National office: (404)816-7800

There are many resources available to you through the American Cancer Society. Free services and products are given through local chapters nationwide and differ from state to state, depending on the financial resources within each particular district. Here are some of the services and products offered:

- Forty hours of home health aide service per year (may be utilized in whatever schedule of days/hours the patient requests).

- One case of Ensure® every other month.

- Transportation to medical appointments for radiation/chemotherapy sessions.

- Free wigs.

- Four psychotherapeutic counseling sessions.

- Support groups.

- Hope Lodges — Lodging for patients and family member during clinical trials.

- Look good...Feel better... — A one-time program for tips on skin care, makeup application, and wig/turban demonstration.

Information on AIDS

- 100 Questions and Answers — Booklet publication by State of New York Department of Health.

- General Information 1-800-541-AIDS
  Spanish Aids Hotline 1-800-233-7432

- Nac Fax — from the Center for Disease Control, National Aids Clearinghouse (1-800-458-5231).

  This is a national reference, referral, and distribution service for HIV/AIDS-related information. To request any materials from the list of available documents, call the above number, and follow instructions. This is a 24 hour fax service.
  FAX (301)738-6616
  Deaf Access 1-800-243-7012

  For more information contact:

  CDC National Aids Clearinghouse
  P.O. Box 6003
  Rockville, MD 20849-6003

Appendix Chapter 7

American Pain Society
5700 Old Country Road
Skokie. IL 60077-1057
(708)966-5595

Booklet: Principles of Analgesic Use in the Treatment of
Acute Pain and Cancer Pain

Agency for Healthcare Policy and Research
Executive Office Center
2101 East Jefferson Street
Suite 501
Rockville, MD 20852

Booklet: *Management of Cancer*
Pain: Adults Quick Reference Guide for Clinicians No. 9

Book: *Clinical Practice Guideline No. 9 Management of
Cancer Pain*. Stock Number 017-022-01182-4
Price: $14.00 (256 pages)
Call (202)512-1800

World Health Organization
Geneva, Switzerland
WWW.who.int

Reports available, Statistics

Safety Data From FDA
WWW.FDA.GOV/CDER/Drug.HTM

Check safety records of particular drugs.

Center Watch
Clinical Trials Listing Service
WWW.Centerwatch.com

Lists more than 7,000 Clinical Trials for treatments and drugs.

IMS HealthInformation
WWW.IMS.Health.Com

Information on prescription drugs.

American Cancer Society
Telephone: 1(800)ACS-2345
WWW.Cancer.org

Information on pain, pain management, pain clinics and programs, and pain specialists.

Mayday Pain Resource Center
City of Hope National Medical Nursing Research and Education
1500 East Duarte Road
Duarte, California 91010
Telephone: (626)359-8111 ext 3829
WWW.Mayday.coh.org

National Cancer Institute
International Cancer Information Center
(800)-4-CANCER
WWW.nci.nih.gov

Commission on Accreditation of Rehabilitation Facilities -
listing of accredited facilities with pain programs
(602)748-1212

Handbook of Cancer Pain Management
from: The Medical College of Wisconsin
and the University of Wisconsin Medical School
in conjunction with the Wisconsin Cancer Pain Initiative
(36 pages) © 1992 (Note: Try contacting the American
Cancer Society for a copy.)

Cancer News on the Net
WWW.cancernews.com

National Cancer Institute's Cancer Net
Cancernet.nci.nih.gov

Oncolink - University of Pennsylvania's Cancer Center
oncolink.upenn.edu

Preferred Rx™
P.O. Box 94863
Cleveland, OH 44101-4863
1(800)677-4323   (216)459-2010   FAX (216)459-2004

Small premium drug plan program for those who do not
have a drug program insurance plan.
• 36,000+ pharmacies nationwide
• Low yearly fee of $20.00 (covers all dependents)
• Discounts of up to 40% off national average
  medication prices
• 100-day supply available
• Mail service
• Dispensing of all FDA approved medication
• Financial hardship waivers
• Plan available for those with or without insurance

VETERANS PROGRAM FOR PRESCRIPTION DRUGS

Call your local veterans administration.

• No cost or for a co-payment of $2.00, depending on
  income

- Yearly enrollment after October 1st
- All veterans over 65 are eligible
- Bring military discharge or separation papers
- Bring financial statement and insurance card
- Physical required at VA (Medicare pays for physical)

Low Income Medication Assistance Programs

A partial list of the free drugs available to low-income patients from the Guide to Low Income Medication Assistance Programs, sponsored by the United States Senate, Special Committee on Aging, Washington, D.C. 20510-6400

Note: The drug companies will only respond to calls from physicians. After you receive the guide, bring it to your physician, or give him or her the number to call.

Drug
BuSpar (antianxiety)
Capoten (Cardiac/antihypertensive)
Cefaclor (antibiotic)
Cefazolln (antibiotic)
Cefzil (antibiotic)
Glipizide (antidiabetic)
Megace (antineoplastic) * also used as an appetite stimulant in patients with AIDS and cancer.
Taxol (antineoplastic)

Company
Bristol-Myers Squibb

Drugs covered: in addition to the drugs listed above, most products manufactured by Bristol-Myers Squibb.
Eligibility: those who are not eligible for prescription drug coverage through their insurance.
Contact: 1-800-736-0003
Bristol-Myers Squibb

Patient Assistance Program
P.O. Box 9445
McLean, VA 22102-9998
* Note - there are many more drugs manufactured by this company that are not included in this list, but are covered in this program.

Drug
Epogen (blood former)
Neupogen (blood former)

Company
Amgen, Inc.
<u>Drugs covered:</u> Epogen, Neupogen
<u>Eligibility:</u> based on income and patient's insurance status.
<u>Contact:</u> 1-800-272-9376 or (202)637-6698

Drug
Darvocet (narcotic analgesic)
Darvon (narcotic analgesic)
Humulin (insulin)
Lletin (insulin)

Company
Eli Lilly

<u>Drugs Covered:</u> in addition to the drugs listed in the left column, most Lilly prescription products and insulins.
<u>Eligibility:</u> determined on case-by-case basis. Based on patient's ability to pay and lack of insurance. Medications are provided to the physician to dispense.
<u>Contact:</u> 1(800)545-6962 Lilly Cares Program Administrator

---

Drug
Duragesic (narcotic analgesic)
Imodium (anti-diarrheal)

Company
Janssen Pharmaceutical
Drugs Covered: Duragesic, Ergamisol, Hismanal, Imodium, Nizoral, Propulsid, Sporanox, Vermox (one or two months supply free)
Eligibility: lack of financial resources and insurance.
Contact: 1(800)544-2987 Janssen Patient Assistant Program 1800 Robert Fulton Drive Reston, Virginia 22091-4346

Drug
Kytril (antiemetic used with chemotherapy)

Company
Smithkline Beecham
Drugs Covered: Kytril, Hycamtin
Eligibility: physician must call on behalf of the patient.
Contact: 1(800)699-3806

Drug
Compazine (antiemetic)

Company
Smithkline Beecham
Eligibility: patient's annual household income is less than $25,000, no insurance, and ineligibility for government or private programs that cover the cost of medications. U.S. resident., a one-time 3 month supply.
Contact: 1(800)546-0420 Access to Care Program
Smithkline Beecham
One Franklin Plaza -FP1320
Philadelphia, Pa 19101

Drug

Oramorph (narcotic analgesic)
Roxanol (narcotic analgesic)
Roxicodone (narcotic analgesic)

Company

Roxanne

<u>Eligibility:</u> product will be provided free of charge to patients through their physician or pharmacist, provided the patient is uninsured and meets annual income requirements. Physicians must call on behalf of the patient.

<u>Contact:</u> 1(800)274-8651

Patient Assistance Program
1101 King Street
Suite 600
Alexandria, VA 22314

U. S. Department of Justice

Drug Enforcement Administration

Office of Diversion Control

Washington, D.C. 20537

Nancy Dahm, R.N., B.S.N.   FEB 0 4 1999

Dear Ms. Dahm:

This is in response to your August 10, 1998 facsimile to Staff Coordinator Larry Houck in which you inquire about the policy of the Drug Enforcement Administration (DEA) on physicians prescribing narcotics for pain management and request government statistics on addiction related to narcotics used for pain management. I apologize for the delay in responding to you.

As you may know, DEA is responsible for enforcing the Controlled Substances Act (CSA), including provisions related to legitimate controlled substances. These provisions exist to ensure that pharmaceutical controlled substances are readily available for legitimate purposes, and also to provide a framework of controls to detect and prevent diversion of these highly abused substances. These medications have legitimate uses and DEA has consistently emphasized and supported a physician's authority to prescribe, dispense or administer them when indicated for a legitimate medical purpose.

The CSA does not set forth standards of medical practice, nor does it limit the quantity of a controlled substance that may be prescribed. It is the responsibility of individual practitioners to treat patients according to their professional judgment in accordance with generally acceptable medical standards. However, physicians also may decide, in their professional judgment, that a patient is abusing or not acting responsibly with a drug. In such instances, a doctor might reduce or stop prescribing for that particular patient.

A physician need not fear DEA action or sanction if he prescribes controlled substances for a legitimate medical purpose within the usual scope of professional practice.

We are in the process of finalizing a policy statement on the use and handling of controlled substances in pain management, which we anticipate will be published in the Federal Register. We will send you a copy of the final policy statement when published. I have, however, enclosed a copy of a speech that I presented to the Federation of State Medical Boards Symposium on Pain Management and State Regulatory Policy in Dallas last March. These remarks further elaborate upon the issue, and recognize recent developments in medical practice standards and treatment modalities.

Nancy Dahm, R.N., B.S.N.   Page 2

Although I am unaware of any comprehensive statistics maintained by DEA which quantify the problem of addiction to pharmaceutical controlled substances, I do know of several examples that indicate the problem's severity. For example, the current street prices of some pharmaceutical drugs, per tablet, include: hydromorphone in Minneapolis for $50, 4 mg. Dilaudid in Knoxville for between $50 and $65, 100 mg. morphine in Louisville for $75, and 8 mg. Dilaudid in Cleveland for between $75 and $100. Additionally, of the top 20 drugs reported by Drug Abuse Warning Network (DAWN) emergency rooms, 12, or 60%, are pharmaceutical controlled substances. Estimates of 1996 emergency room estimates include 15,247 alprazolam episodes, 14,911 unspecified benzodiazepine episodes, 13,089 diazepam episodes, 12,699 clonazepam episodes, 10,248 hydrocodone episodes, 9,491 lorazepam episodes, 8,952 amphetamine episodes, 6,449 d-propoxyphene episodes, 6,440 codeine combination episodes, 3,810 methadone episodes, and 3,012 oxycodone episodes. I suggest that you contact the United States Food and Drug Administration (FDA) and the Office of National Drug Control Policy for additional information.

I hope that this information is useful to you. If you have any additional inquiries, please do not hesitate to contact Staff Coordinator Houck of my staff at (202) 307-7286.

Sincerely,

Patricia M. Good, Chief
Liaison and Policy Section

Enclosure

cc: DPM Margaret A. Brophy, New York Division
      G/S Robert Brown, Long Island District Office

PAIN SCALE FLOW SHEET (0-10 SCALE)

Current Analgesic Prescribed

Doctor   Phone Number

SIDE EFFECTS TO BE REPORTED IMMEDIATELY

DA = Difficult to Arouse   N =Nausea   V =Vomiting   C = Constipation

DATE	TIME	PAIN RATING	MEDICATION CHANGE	RESP/PULSE	SIDE EFFECTS /COMMENTS

Appendix Chapter 9

Corporate Angel Network, Inc.
Westchester County Airport
One Loop Road
White Plains, New York 10604
(914)328-1313
website:www.Corporateangelnetwork.org.

This is a non-for-profit organization that helps cancer patients fly free for recognized cancer treatment. Requests can be taken up to three weeks in advance. Travel may be as often as necessary, and the patient may fly with an adult companion. Certain qualifications apply:

• The need to travel for treatment, consultation, or check-up.

• Able to walk up the stairs of a private jet without assistance.

• Requiring no form of life support or medical help on board.

On-line Resources - Clinical Trials

American Medical Association
http://www.ama.assn.org.
Clinical trials, resources, HIV/AIDS.

Cancer Care's Clinical Trials Resources
http://www.cancercareinc.org/help/clinical.htm
General information about clinical trials.

Cancer Web
cancerweb@www.graylab.ac.uk

Center Watch Clinical Trials Listing
http://www.centerwatch.com

The Brain Tumor Society
http://www.tbts.org

Kimmel Cancer Center: Clinical Trials
http://www.jci.tju.edu

National Cancer Institute's CancerNet
http://cancernet.nci.nih.gov

NCI and NABCO: Breast Cancer Trial Directory
http://www.nabco.org

National Institutes of Health Sponsored Clinical Trials
http://medoc.gdb.org/best/fedfund/nih-select/clinical.html

National Institutes of Health and FDA database information on clinical trials.
http://www.clinicaltrials.gov

Oncolink: Clinical Trials News
http://cancer.med.upenn.edu/upcc/clin_trials

Sterling Clinical Resources
http://clinical-trials.com

Appendix Chapter 11
ENTERAL NUTRITIONALS
APPLICATION FOR ASSISTANCE
(To Be Completed by Physician)

PATIENT'S NAME _____

ADDRESS _____

_____

_____

_____ TELEPHONE _____

DIAGNOSIS _____

_____

PRODUCT _____

AMOUNT USED PER DAY _____

FLAVORS PREFERRED _____

DURATION ON PRODUCT _____

FINANCIAL INFORMATION (Include why patient is seeking assistance;

insurance coverage, work situation, etc):

APPROXIMATE MONTHLY INCOME NEEDED

_____

_____

DOCTOR'S NAME _____

ADDRESS _____

_____

_____

SIGNATURE _____

DATE _____ TELEPHONE _____

RETURN COMPLETED FORM TO: MEAD JOHNSON NUTRITIONALS

CONSUMER AFFAIRS - F21

ALL SECTIONS MUST BE COMPLETED!!   2400 W. LLOYD EXPRESSWAY

EVANSVILLE, IN 47721

FAX TO: (812)423-8583 OR CONTACT 1-800-247-7893 BETWEEN THE

HOURS OF 1:00 TO 4:00 PM CENTRAL TIME.

STATE OF NEW YORK
DEPARTMENT OF HEALTH

Nonhospital Order Not to Resuscitate (DNR Order)

Person's Name _____

Date of Birth ____/____/____

Do not resuscitate the person named above.

Physician's Signature _____

Print Name _____

License Number _____

Date ____/____/____

It is the responsibility of the physician to determine, at least every 90 days, whether this order continues to be appropriate, and to indicate this by a note in the person's medical chart.   The issuance of a new form is NOT required and under the law this order should be considered valid unless it is known that it has been revoked. This order remains valid and must be followed, even if it has not been reviewed within the 90 day period.

REFERENCES

1 Agency for the Health Care Policy and Research. *Management of Cancer Pain: Adults.* ACHPR Pub. No. 94-0592, 1994.

2 Brumbaugh, Robert. *The Philosophers of Greece.* New York: State University of New York Press, 1981.

3 Connolly, John and Castle, John. *The Castle Connolly Guide to the ABC's of HMO's: How to Get the Best From Managed Care.* New York: Castle Connolly Medical Ltd. 1997.

4 Eliot, Charles W. *The Harvard Classics.* Connecticut: Grolier, 1980.

5 Friedman, D.P., *Perspectives on Medical Use of Drugs of Abuse.* Journal of Pain Symptom Management 5:S2-S5, Feb. 1990.

6 Goldberg, R.J. and Tull, R.M. *The Psychological Dimensions of Cancer.* New York: MacMillan, 1994.

7 Guyton, Arthur C. *Textbook of Medical Physiology.* 9th ed. Philadelphia: W.B. Saunders Company, 1995.

8 Hogan, Catherine M. and Wickman, Rita. *Issues in Managing the Oncology Patient.* New York: Philips Healthcare Communication, Inc., 1996.

9 Jacox A, Carr DB, Payne R, et al. *The Management of Cancer Pain.* Clinical practice guideline number 9. AHCPR Publication No. 94-0592. Rockville, Md.: Agency for Health Care Policy and Research, U.S. Department of Health and Human Services, Public Health Service, 1994.

10 Johnson, Barbara Schoen. *Psychiatric Mental Health Nursing: Adaptation and Growth,.* 2nd ed. New York: Lippincott, 1989.

11   Lefrancois, Guy. *The Life Span*. California: Wadsworth, 1993.

12   Melling. David. *Understanding Plato*. New York: Oxford University Press, 1987.

13   Nicoli, Armand. *The New Harvard Guide to Psychiatry*. Massachusetts: Belknap Press, 1988.

14   Porter, J. and Jick, H.: *"Addiction rare in patients treated with Narcotics."* N. Eng. J. Med., 302 (1980): 123.

15   Portnoy, RK., McCaffrey, M.: *Adjuvant-analgesics*. In: McCaffrey, M., Pasero, C.: *Pain: Clinical Manual*. St. Louis: Mosby Inc., 1999.

16   Rodwell, Williams, Sue. *Nutrition and Diet Therapy*. 6th ed. St. Louis: Mosby College Publishing, 1989.

17   Spradley, Barbara Walton and Allender, Judith Ann. *Community Health Nursing: Concepts and Practice*. New York: Lippincott, 1996.

18   Spradley, Barbara Walton. *Readings in Community Health Nursing*. New York: J.B. Lippincott Company, 1991.

19   Strong, B. *"The View from the Mattress"* Nursing 92. (May 1992): 47-49.

20   Tortora, Gerard J. and Anagnostakos. *Principles of Anatomy and Physiology*. New York: Harper and Row, 1987.

21   World Health Organization. *Making Opiod's Available to Treat Cancer Pain: The International System*. Vol. 7, No. 2-3, 1994.

A